MEDITERRANEAN DIET COOKBOOK FOR BEGINNERS

101 Quick and Healthy Recipes with Easy-to-Find Ingredients to Enjoy The Mediterranean Lifestyle

SANDRA COOK

ENJOY THE MEDITERRANEAN LIFESTYLE

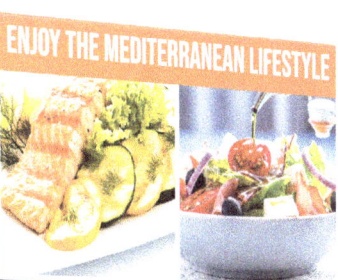

EASY-TO-FIND INGREDIENTS

MEDITERRANEAN DIET COOKBOOK FOR BEGINNERS

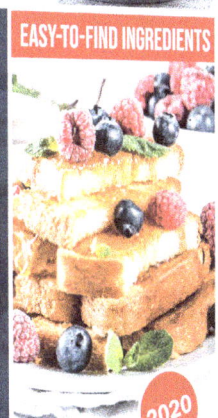

2020

21-DAY MEAL PLAN TO WEIGHT LOSS

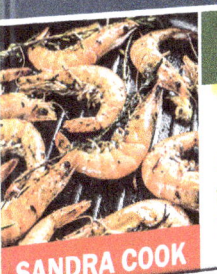
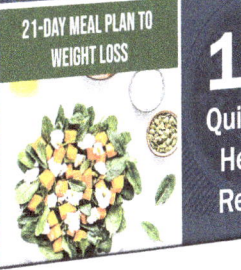

101 Quick and Healthy Recipes

SANDRA COOK

Copyright © 2020 by Sandra Cook

All rights reserved

No part of this guide may be reproduced in any form without permission in writing from the publisher except in the case of brief quotations embodied in critical articles or reviews.

Legal & Disclaimer

The information contained in this book and its contents is not designed to replace or take the place of any form of medical or professional advice; and is not meant to replace the need for independent medical, financial, legal or other professional advice or services, as may be required. The content and information in this book has been provided for educational and entertainment purposes only.

The content and information contained in this book has been compiled from sources deemed reliable, and it is accurate to the best of the Author's knowledge, information and belief. However, the Author cannot guarantee its accuracy and validity and cannot be held liable for any errors and/or omissions. Further, changes are periodically made to this book as and when needed. Where appropriate and/or necessary, you must consult a professional (including but not limited to your doctor, attorney, financial advisor or such other professional advisor) before using any of the suggested remedies, techniques, or information in this book.

Upon using the contents and information contained in this book, you agree to hold harmless the Author from and against any damages, costs, and expenses, including any legal fees potentially resulting from the application of any of the information provided by this book. This disclaimer applies to any loss, damages or injury caused by the use and application, whether directly or indirectly, of any advice or information presented, whether for breach of contract, tort, negligence, personal injury, criminal intent, or under any other cause of action.

You agree to accept all risks of using the information presented inside this book. You agree that by continuing to read this book, where appropriate and/or necessary, you shall consult a professional (including but not limited to your doctor, attorney, or financial advisor or such other advisor as needed) before using any of the suggested remedies, techniques, or information in this book.

CONTENTS

Preface	ix
Introduction	xv
1. The Incredible Health Benefits	1
2. Path To Weight Loss	7
3. The Mediterranean Diet Pyramid	10
4. Your Mediterranean Diet Shopping List	13
5. Fundamentals	21
6. Essential Nutrients & Food Sources	29
7. Getting Started	32
8. How to Manage Portions?	39

Part One
BREAKFAST

Breakfast Quesadilla	45
Hearty Breakfast Frittata w/ Tomato Salad	48
Spaghetti Frittata	50
Chickpea & Potato Hash	53
Mediterranean Breakfast Quinoa	55
Breakfast Enchiladas	57
Mediterranean Breakfast Wraps	60
Panera Mediterranean Breakfast Sandwich	63
Greek Scramble	65
Cheesy Mediterranean Scramble	67
Mediterranean Omelet	69
Huevos Revueltos	71
Creamy Cuban Fu Fu	73
Roasted Asparagus Prosciutto & Egg	75
Creamy Loaded Mashed Potatoes	78
Potato and Zucchini Omelet	80
Secret Breakfast Sundaes	83
Banana Nut Oatmeal	85
Greek Frittata w/ Zucchini, Tomatoes, Feta, and Herbs	87

Greek Yogurt Pancakes	90
Mediterranean Tofu Scramble	92

Part Two
LUNCH

Smoked Salmon and Veggies Mix	97
Salmon and Creamy Endives	99
Baked Trout and Fennel	101
Lamb Steak Pita Breads	103
Baked Lamb with Eggplant and Greek Yogurt	105
Beef Steaks with Spicy Sauce	108
Delicious Sausage Kebabs	111
Turkey Cutlets	114
Slow Cooked Chicken	117
Mediterranean Meatloaf	120
Chili Calamari and Veggie Mix	123
Greek Trout Spread	125
Cayenne Cod and Tomatoes	127
Shrimp and Dill Mix	129
Salmon & Asparagus	131
High-Quality Belizean Chicken Stew	133
The Great Poblano Chicken Curry	135
The Original Mexican Chicken Cacciatore	137
Magnificent Chicken Curry Soup	139
Awesome Ligurian Chicken	141
Garlic And Lemon Chicken Dish	144

Part Three
DINNER

Garlic Shrimp with Olive Oil	149
Steamed Mussels in Tomato Garlic	151
Mediterranean-style Mussels	153
Leeks and Calamari Mix	155
Seafood Paella	157
Baked Salmon in Garlic Pepper	159
Sauteed Octopus	162
Grilled Octopus	164
Scallop Salad	166
Delicious Chicken Soup	169

Classic Mediterranean Chicken Soup	172
Easy Chicken Stew	175
Chicken and Cabbage Mix	177
Mediterranean Chicken and Rice Soup	179
Healthy Mediterranean Chicken	181
Mushroom And Chicken Bowl	183
Chicken And Broccoli Platter	185
Daring Salted Baked Chicken	188
Worthy Ghee-Licious Chicken	190
Chicken Korma	192
Turkey With Garlic Sauce	194

Part Four
SNACKS & DESSERTS

Healthy Coconut Blueberry Balls	199
Crunchy Roasted Chickpeas	201
Tasty Zucchini Chips	203
Roasted Green Beans	205
Savory Pistachio Balls	207
Roasted Almonds	209
Banana Strawberry Popsicles	211
Chocolate Matcha Balls	213
Chia Almond Butter Pudding	215
Refreshing Strawberry Popsicles	217
Dark Chocolate Mousse	219
Warm & Soft Baked Pears	221
Healthy & Quick Energy Bites	223
Creamy Yogurt Banana Bowls	225
Chocolate Mousse	227
Carrot Spread	230
Chicken Wings Platter	232
Stuffed Chicken	234
Cinnamon Baby Back Ribs Platter	236
Buttery Carrot Sticks	238
Cajun Walnuts And Olives Bowls	240
Mango Salsa	242
Hot Asparagus Sticks	244
Pork Bites	246

Part Five
SALADS & SIDE DISHES

Tender Roasted Sweet Potatoes with Savory Tahini Sauce	251
Homemade Whole Wheat Pita Bread	253
Crisp Spiced Cauliflower with Feta Cheese	256
Spring Peas and Beans with Zesty Thyme Yogurt Sauce	258
Mediterranean Pasta Salad	261
Mediterranean Farro Salad	263
Mediterranean Couscous	266
Loaded Mediterranean Cauliflower Fries	268
Mediterranean Succotash	271
Mediterranean Couscous Salad	273
Mediterranean Barley Salad	276
Tabbouleh	279
Spinach Salad with Grilled Mediterranean Vegetables	281
Mediterranean Chicken Samosas with Apple Cumin Chutney	283
Toasted Israeli Couscous with Vegetables and Lemon-Balsamic Vinaigrette	286
Elbow Macaroni with Pine Nuts, Lemon and Fennel	289
Vegetable Couscous	292
Saffron Rice Salad	295
Lemon Rice	297
Carrot Slaw	299
Greek Salad with Saganaki	301
21-Day Meal Plan	305
Conclusion	319
Final Words	321
Measurement Conversions	323
References	327
Index Recipes	329

PREFACE

Thank you for downloading this book. The reason why I created this cookbook is to get you started on your new healthy lifestyle. If is it true that we are what we eat, then this lifestyle transformation needs to start from our plates and my promise is to help you stay committed with delicious and mouthwatering Mediterranean recipes that are quick and easy to prepare.

My name is Sandra, I am an Italian chef and author with a great passion for healthy food. With the help of my friend, Sara Scotti, who is a nutritionist, we have been able to plan one of the healthiest meal plan which in 21 days only, will introduce you into the Mediterranean lifestyle. Together as a team, we researched and outlined 101 vibrant recipes to make sure you are getting all the right foods in your body at just the right time of the day. This involves the right combination of meats, fish, carbs, fats, fruit and vegetables. Also, we added lots of delicious snacks and desserts in the mix as bonus!

All the recipes in this cookbook are **kitchen-tested** and are designed to help you to easily follow the Mediterranean diet daily, with a lot of **tips and science-based information** to improve your health. To make all this easier, **each recipe is accompanied by a nutritional analysis and a photo** showing the final result.

Often, a lot of clients ask me " What is the difference between success and failure in Mediterranean diet?"

Well, the key to succeeding on any diet is to have a plan, for the Mediterranean diet is the same. Most people on a new diet have no plan. They learn what to eat and not to eat, they try new recipes, but they do not have a daily plan to carry them through the critical first month.

Without a plan, it's very easy to fall for peer pressure, to be unprepared, and to make bad decisions.

Hence, the reason we have created this **foolproof 21-day diet program** to help you through your Mediterranean diet journey.

If you have ever been on a diet before, you would know just how hard it is to figure out what you can and can't eat, plan your meals, keep track of your calories, make room for just enough dessert, manage your diet with your busy schedule and stay motivated.

Here's the difference! We have done all this work(**and tested,** also) to make things easier for you.

This means you will know exactly when and what to eat without having to second guess yourself.

Here's what you will get:

- Guidelines for eating the Mediterranean way, as well as tips to improve your health and (if you desire) maximize your weight loss.
- Easy-to-find ingredients from your local grocery store and tips for your shopping list.
- 101 insanely delicious recipes that focus on whole foods, structured upon the Mediterranean pyramid.
- A 21-day adventure of trying and preparing new dishes without spending hours in the kitchen or googling recipes.
- Nutritional information with recipe instructions on the best food sources.

- Science-based insights behind the Mediterranean fundamentals like olive oil and red wine.
- Best tips to integrate the Mediterranean diet into your life and the main 8 factors to stick to it.

Now, stop talking... it's time to start this flavourful and healthiest journey into the Mediterranean Lifestyle!

"The doctor of the future will no longer treat human frame with drugs, but rather will cure and prevent disease with nutrition."
   -Thomas Edison

INTRODUCTION

The Mediterranean Diet is a nutritional model and a lifestyle inspired by the habits of countries all around the Mediterranean sea. Interests in this diet began in the 1960s, thanks to Ancel Keys, an American biologist and physiologist, who discovered the link between eating habits and the health benefits of local populations. His contributions has helped in birthing the famous volume *"Eat Well and Stay Well"*.

According to researchers, communities living along the Mediterranean have exceptionally low risk regarding lifestyle diseases compared to people from other Western countries. Numerous studies have been conducted and they all show that the Mediterranean diet is beneficial to our health and wellbeing. Observing this diet regularly will help prevent health conditions such as strokes, heart attacks, type II diabetes, as well as premature death.

The World's Healthiest Diet

The **WHO (World Health Organization agency)** recognized the Mediterranean diet as one of the healthiest diets in the world and it is also recommended by the **Dietary Guidelines for Americans**. The rating is mainly because of the kinds of foods obtainable in this region. This diet is built on daily exercise along with a lot of fruit, vegetables, plant-based proteins, whole grains, fish and smaller amounts of poultry, red meat and simple sugars. Fatty fish (salmon), olive oil, and nuts make this diet higher in fat than the classic "heart-healthy diet." These fats are mostly "healthy fats" and are also called monounsaturated fats. When consumed in the right proportion, these fats are good for the heart.

While the Mediterranean diet is not your typical run-of-the-mill diet, it is actually a lifestyle. You can think of it as a different way of eating and living. Following this lifestyle, you can make well-balanced food choices that boost your health and taste great while promoting weight loss and development of lean muscle.

Key Components of the Mediterranean Diet

If you wish to follow the Mediterranean diet lifestyle, then you need to understand its key components.

These include the following:

- Eating mostly plant-based foods such as green leafy vegetables, fruits, and whole grains.
- Replacing butter and margarine with healthy oils like olive oil.
- Making use of spices and herbs for flavouring rather than salt.
- Eating moderate portions of poultry and eggs once a week or every two days.
- Limiting your intake of red meats to either weekends or a couple of times per month. You can also limit red meat consumption to three-ounce portions.
- Eating fish or fish products at least two times weekly.
- Having moderate sizes of yogurt and cheese daily, every other day or weekly.
- Drinking a lot of water each day.
- Drink some red wine but in moderation.
- Physical activity.

Chapter One
THE INCREDIBLE HEALTH BENEFITS

LOWERS RISK OF CARDIOVASCULAR DISEASE

The Mediterranean diet has been recognized to be most helpful in reducing high triglyceride levels. Triglycerides are fatty molecules that travel throughout the bloodstream and build up plaque in our arteries. A higher triglyceride count or its accumulation in the bloodstream and vessels can lead to higher cholesterol and an increased risk of stroke or heart attack. Even though the Mediterranean diet consists of fatty items like olive oil and salmon, they are good fats that are loaded with beneficial monounsaturated and polyunsaturated fats.

A study carefully tracked and analyzed 28 men who ate Mediterranean diet meals, followed by junk food meals for a week. They found that after the men had the Mediterranean meal, their arteries opened and they maintained a healthy blood flow. This was compared to after the junk food meal when their arteries failed to dilate and their blood flow function did not improve.

The Mediterranean diet proves more effective at reducing high triglyceride counts, while still maintaining the presence of "good" cholesterol (or HDL cholesterol) in the blood.

. . .

IMPROVES HEART HEALTH

The study shows that a Mediterranean diet rich in ALA (alpha-linolenic acid) found in olive oil can decrease the risk of cardiac death in a person by nearly 30. Further research shows that when comparing the blood pressure between people who consumed sunflower oil versus those consuming extra virgin oil, the olive oil consumers were able to decrease their blood pressure by more significant amounts.

It might seem counterintuitive that olive oil can actually lower blood pressure, but the peculiarity of virgin olive oil is to be an unrefined oil, which means that the plant additions are intact and can improve cellular function. By adding this with the healthy fats consumed in the Mediterranean diet, it will surely allow your body to slowly decrease the amount of unhealthy triglycerides you are consuming to improve overall heart health.

WEIGHT LOSS

The types of food that the Mediterranean diet encourages such as whole grains, beans, and legumes, contain high amounts of fiber, which help to slow digestion and prevent frequent spikes in blood sugar levels. That means you feel full for a longer period without needing a snack.

Blood sugar spikes are dangerous to our body because in order to contrast them, the body is forced to produce high amounts of insulin, a hormone that causes weight gain. Also, fibers in contact with water become swollen and contribute to an increased satiety, thereby preventing you from eating more food than necessary.

Mediterranean diet is less caloric than the fatty diet of many western countries, and it makes a large use of aromatic herbs that allow you to flavour the dishes, which has little or no amounts of fatty and high-calorie condiments.

CAN HELP TO FIGHT CANCER

Of course, there's no cure for cancer, but studies have found that the Mediterranean diet provides the most favorable conditions for the body to fight against cancer. A 2013 study at the University of Genoa in Italy found that the Mediterranean diet provides your body with a balanced ratio of omega fatty acids, fiber, and antioxidants found in wine, fruits, vegetables, and olive oil. Providing high amounts of antioxidants is the key in fighting cancer cells and stopping further cell mutation.

A study at the Mayo Clinic found that 800 people with advanced colon polyps ate red meat more frequently and their diet did not correspond to foods on the Mediterranean diet. The World Cancer Research Fund reports that eating at least 90 grams of whole grains a day can reduce your risk of colon cancer by almost 20%. This is because the fiber in whole grains prevents any mutations from developing in your digestive tract and keeps your bowel movement in check.

Protects Cognitive Health

Following the Mediterranean diet could be key in protecting yourself from future neurodegenerative diseases like Parkinson's, dementia, or Alzheimer's. The healthy fats that the Mediterranean diet is full of are known to fight age-related cognitive decline, along with the anti-inflammatory protection that fresh fruits and vegetables provide.

The Taub Institute for Research in Alzheimer's Disease found that the more strictly the individuals in their test group followed the Mediterranean diet, the lower their risk for developing Alzheimer's disease. Doctors have always encouraged seniors and patients at risk for neurodegenerative diseases to adopt healthier eating habits to possibly delay or inhibit their symptoms of dementia. Following a Mediterranean diet can improve your memory, mental acuity, and attention span as it protects your nerve cells from deteriorating with age.

Increase Your Lifespan!

A famous research called the Lyon Diet Heart Study tested a group of individuals who had heart attacks between 1988 and 1992. They were counseled to follow a traditional post-heart attack diet or the Mediterranean diet.

When a follow-up study was conducted after 4 years, the results found that the people following the Mediterranean diet had a reduced risk of heart disease by 70%. They also experienced a nearly 50% lower risk of death than the standard low-fat diet. It seems that the combination of fresh fruits and vegetables in addition to healthy fat sources like beans, nuts, and fish are a winning combination to extend the human lifespan.

Protection Against Type-2 Diabetes

With the Mediterranean diet, you limit yourself to eat less processed foods and the fat your body absorbs are mostly from olive oil, nuts, and healthy meats. It's not a "low carb" diet, but still reduces the amount of your carbohydrate intake, so that fewer carbs are converted to glucose. A 2011 study in Spain discovered that after a 4-year research, participants assigned to a Mediterranean style diet had a reduced risk of developing Type 2 diabetes by more than 50%. The result showed that there was a massive progress compared to the other group that followed a low-fat diet.

The Mediterranean diet encourages meals seasoned with healthy spices, and also encourages you to fill your dessert with fruit instead of baked foods that contain sugar. It is also important to note that in many studies, participants on the Mediterranean diet tended to lose on average more weight than participants on other low carb or low-fat diets. Due to this weight loss, you can reduce your risk of diabetes, and maybe even delay needing any further medication.

Improves Sex Life

Erectile dysfunction or ED is a common side effect of cardiovascular disease. As the blood vessels are blocked with unhealthy plaque, the smaller vessels leading towards the male genitalia are unable to respond like they used to. But research shows that the Mediterranean diet can help with this too!

A study in Italy tested a group of nearly 70 men by putting half on a control diet and another half on a Mediterranean diet. After two years of study, more than one-third of the men who followed the Mediterranean diet strictly regained normal sexual functioning. Though there's no exact reason for this, as it is believed that the fiber and healthy antioxidants in fresh fruits and vegetables can promote blood flow throughout the body.

Increase Sight

Since the Mediterranean diet is full of fruits, vegetables, and regular servings of fish, it has great amounts of vitamins that protect your sight. According to the American Academy of Ophthalmology, eye health is protected by eating antioxidants which are found in fresh plant products. Fish is also high in omega 3 fatty acids which is critical to sight health. Just having one serving of fish in a week can lower the risk of developing eye damage which occurs commonly in people over the age of 50. With the Mediterranean diet, you are incorporating fish in your diet more than two times a week! The seeds and nuts you are eating as snacks also contain fatty acids that protect the retinas from cellular damage, which occurs with age.

Your Kidney Function Improves

Your kidneys are constantly working throughout the day to filter waste and liquid from your body while still maintaining your blood pressure. But chronic kidney disease can affect more than 30 million Americans a year.

A 2014 study in the ***Clinical Journal of American Society of Nephrology*** found that following the Mediterranean diet may decrease the chances of having chronic kidney disease by almost 50%. This could be attributed to clean and healthy food choices that the Mediterranean diet requires, with less processed food and red meat. Fish, nuts, fresh fruits and vegetables are known to lower inflammation in the body, which causes kidney disease.

. . .

KEEPS YOUR SKIN HEALTHY

A diet rich in antioxidants found in fresh fruits and vegetables helps to keep your skin at its healthiest. That means a healthy growth, strong elasticity, and prevention against common skin conditions like eczema, acne, or rosacea. One of the worst foods for your skin is sugar, which can cause inflammation in our body, thus contributing to the breakdown of collagen, a helpful protein that keeps the skin firm.

By following the Mediterranean diet, you will cut out extra sugar and instead rely on healthy fruits with natural sugars. A study even found that people with higher blood sugar levels were considered "older-looking" based on the appearance of their skin compared to people with low blood sugar levels. Eating a balanced diet full of healthy vitamins and minerals keeps your skin healthy and that's exactly what the Mediterranean diet provides!

PROTECT THE BODY FROM STRESS AND AGING

Studies conducted by a team of researchers from the University of Milan and Parma show that the Mediterranean diet reduces inflammation in the body and also helps to protect the body against oxidative stress. Most of the foods present in the Mediterranean diet represent a rich source of bioactive compounds such as vitamins, carotenoids, glucosinolates and polyphenols that act as antioxidants or endogenous multiple defense systems activators.

The research led to the conclusion that the Mediterranean Diet plays a key role in protecting DNA damage and modulating DNA repair genes and telomere length, which means you can feel the benefits of healthy skin, more energy, and longevity of your cells, especially the nerve cells that keeps your brain active and functioning at top mental acuity.

Chapter Two
PATH TO WEIGHT LOSS

If you are interested in applying the Mediterranean diet to lose weight, then these general dieting tips paired with a healthier lifestyle will help you maximize your weight loss.

EAT SLOWLY

It takes twenty minutes for your food to start digesting and give you a feeling of fullness after ingesting a meal. Therefore, slow down and chew your food so that you can actually taste it and enjoy the flavour. If you tend to eat fast, you may find that you eat more because it takes that twenty minutes to get your internal system all fired up.

DRINK WATER BEFORE YOUR MEAL

Try drinking a full eight-ounce glass of water before you sit down to eat a meal. Sometimes thirst can be mistaken for the feeling of hunger. Drinking a glass of water before you eat can get the digestion process to start quicker, which can cause you to eat less during a meal.

. . .

Manage portions

Visually split your plate in half, then split one of those halves in two. This makes three sections....two small ones and one big one.

The big section should be for vegetables and the two smaller sections are for your whole grains and proteins. You can use this as a measuring guide when you go out to eat or want to transition your dinner plate into healthier portions.

You will receive the highest levels of phytonutrients from vegetables, and that is the reason vegetables should occupy the largest section of the plate.

Exercise

Physical activity is one of the fundamental "ingredients" for weight loss. By simply reducing your calorie intake without increasing movement, you risk losing muscle mass.

Adhere to the lowest, most foundational level of the Mediterranean pyramid which is a daily activity. Do your best to get 30 minutes of exercise every day.

Change the way you think about food

See vegetables and fruits as snacks. Slice your vegetables into ready to eat snack sizes and wash your fruits when you bring them home from the store. Then make ready to grab as a quick snack when you are feeling hungry.

Keep a jar of mixed nuts on your kitchen counter and eat a handful of those along with your vegetable or fruit snack.

Pre Packaged snacks

Pre Packaged snacks into portion sizes rather than eating from the full container. Doing this can prevent overeating. When you pre-allocate how much of a snack you're going to eat, then you are helping yourself stay disciplined.

. . .

SNACK TWO OR THREE TIMES A DAY

Enjoy two or three snacking times a day where you eat a serving of fruit or vegetables with no salt or sugar added. Schedule a snack in the morning, afternoon and before going to bed.

REPLACE CAKES AND COOKIES

Replace frequent cake and cookie binges with a serving of popcorn cooked in olive oil and sprinkled with parmesan cheese or garlic powder rather than salt and butter.

BUY SMALLER PLATES AND BOWLS

When you fill up a smaller plate or bowl, you can still get the satisfaction of having a full plate or bowl. When your plate or bowl is smaller, you can feel satisfied but still be able to eat in healthy portions that adhere to the pyramid.

REPLACE SATURATED FATS WITH MONOUNSATURATED FATS

Give your weight loss program the super-charged fuel it needs by replacing your saturated fats with monounsaturated fats. The Mediterranean diet replaces a standard bad fat diet with high levels of healthy monounsaturated fats that raises good cholesterol levels.

LEARN A WELL-BALANCED EATING PLAN

The longer you adhere to the Mediterranean diet, the more energy and vitality you will experience.

The 21-day Mediterranean diet offers exactly a well-balanced eating plan that includes the correct amount of each food group.

Chapter Three
THE MEDITERRANEAN DIET PYRAMID

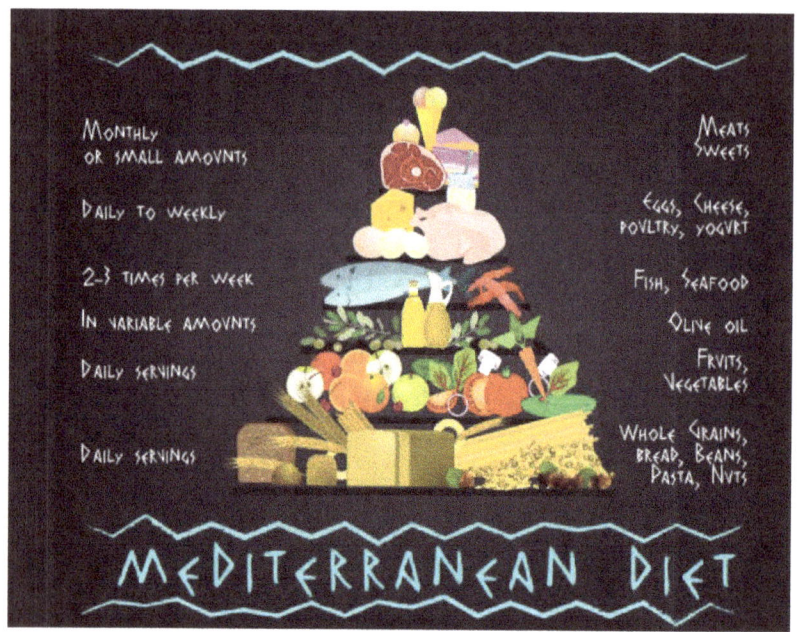

The Mediterranean Diet Pyramid is a nutritional guide that was developed by Oldways Preservation Trust, the World Health Organization and by the Harvard School of Public Health in 1993. It is a visual tool that summarizes the Mediterranean diet suggested pattern of eating and gives a guide to how frequently specific tools should be eaten. This allows you to have a breakdown of healthy eating habits and not to overfill yourself with too many calories.

How is the pyramid laid out? Let's go over each tier.

Olive oil, fruits, vegetables, whole grains, legumes, beans, nuts & seeds, spices & herbs: These food form the base of the Mediterranean pyramid. If you did observe, you will notice that these are mostly from plant sources. You should try and include a few variations of these items into each meal you eat. Olive oil should be the main fat in cooking your dishes and endeavour to replace any other butter or cooking oil you may have been using to cook.

Generous uses of herbs and spices are also encouraged to season your food and add flavor as an alternative to salt. If you don't have access to fresh herbs, you can buy the dried version. This will serve as well. Always be sure to read the nutrition labels to ensure there are no other ingredients mixed with the herbs. Fresh ginger, garlic and onion are also great flavor enhancers for your meals. They can be easily stored in the freezer.

Fish & seafood: These are important staples of the Mediterranean diet that should be consumed often as a protein source. You would want to include these in your diet for at least two times a week. Try new varieties of fish, either frozen or fresh. Also incorporate seafood like mussels, crab, and shrimp into your diet. Canned tuna is also great to include on sandwiches or toss in a salad with fresh vegetables.

Cheese, yogurt, eggs & poultry: These ingredients should be consumed in more moderate amounts. Depending on the food, they should be used sparingly throughout the week. Keep in mind that if you are using eggs in baking or cooking, they will also be counted in your weekly limit. You would want to stick to more healthy cheese like Parmesan, ricotta, or feta that you can add as a topping or garnish on your dishes.

Red meat & sweets: These items are going to be consumed less frequently. If you are going to eat them, then you need to be sure to consume only small quantities, most preferably lean meat versions with less fat when possible. Most studies recommend a maximum of 12 to 16 ounces per month. To add some variety to your diet, You can still have red meat occasionally but you would want to reduce how often you have it. It is important to limit its intake because of all the health concerns that come with sugar and red meat. The Mediterranean diet is working to improve cardiovascular health and reduce blood pressure, while red meat tends to be dangerous to your cardiovascular system. The Greece population ate very little red meat and instead had fish or seafood as their main source of protein.

Water: The Mediterranean diet encourages you to stay hydrated at all times. This means drinking more water than your daily intake. The Institute of Medicine recommends a total of 9 cups each day for women and 13 cups for men. For a pregnant or breastfeeding woman, the number should be increased.

Wine: Moderate consumption of wine with meals is encouraged on the Mediterranean diet. Studies have shown that moderate consumption of alcohol can reduce the risk of heart disease. That can mean about 1 glass per day for women. Men tend to have higher body mass, so they can consume 1 to 2 glasses. Please keep in mind what your doctor would recommend regarding wine consumption based on your health and family history.

Chapter Four

YOUR MEDITERRANEAN DIET SHOPPING LIST

To make it easier for you, we have suggestions of what exactly you need to include on your shopping list to follow the Mediterranean diet! We will let you know what you need to include and what you need to leave out.

Include:

- ***Extra virgin and virgin olive oils***: These are the least processed and refined versions of olive oil in the market (best labeled as EVOO - extra virgin olive oil). They contain the highest level of plant compounds called "phenols" that act as antioxidants in the body. It might be a little pricier than the oil you used before, but it's well worth it when you are aware of the health benefits you will gain by using it! This will be your go-to oil when it comes to cooking, frying, seasoning, and as the base of your salad dressings. Remember, less is more!
- ***Fish & Seafood***: Whether it's mackerel, trout, sardines,

tuna, salmon, or tilapia, fish is going to be a staple for you on the Mediterranean diet! These types of fatty fish are rich sources of omega 3 fatty acids throughout the week. Be sure to experiment with new types so you don't get tired of the same one! You can even use canned fish like sardines or anchovies because cured fish was very common in Greece. Try and look for the low sodium versions to avoid excess salt intake. Don't forget to add shrimp, crab, or mussels so you can expand your seafood palate!

- **Vegetables:** You have pretty much free rein with vegetables if you can stick to low-calorie ones, as it's best for your weight loss goals. Vegetables like zucchini, mushrooms, cabbage, cauliflower, bell pepper, and spinach are low in calories but are still very filling and high in fiber. Try new vegetables and eating them in different ways like steamed, sautèd, grilled or different salad combinations, so you don't get bored eating them. Try to buy in season items so you can save yourself some money!

- **Fruits:** Fruits are encouraged and are great as a substitute healthy dessert. Figs and pomegranates are native to the Mediterranean area, but any fruit will do! Be sure to include a variety of colourful fruits and vegetables which allows you to have a diverse range of essential vitamins and minerals. If you are diabetic, try and consume fruits that are low on the glycemic index such as oranges, apples, grapefruits, pears, or plums.

- **Legumes & beans:** These are a great hidden source of protein that often get overlooked in the West in favour of red meat or poultry items. Thankfully, the Mediterranean diet urges you to try different variations of protein sources! Whether it's black beans, kidney beans, chickpeas, or lentils, they are all great to experiment with. Don't forget hummus! These are packed with fiber as well, so they allow you to feel full for a longer period. Be sure you drink plenty of water to avoid constipation!

- ***Whole grain breads and cereal:*** Whether it's rice, barley, oats, leek rice, quinoa, whole grain pasta, or whole grain bread, you would want to be sure you are focused on whole grains that are healthier rather than refined or processed grains. The same goes with cereal. Be sure you read the label and ensure that the product is made from whole grain starches and are not processed into refined products. Ezekiel bread is a whole grain bread made with no sugar. One slice is packed with fiber and contains only 80 calories! The trick with whole grains is that you can eat a smaller portion than you would with refined wheat products, but you will stay full for a longer period. They are also low on the glycemic index scale which makes them safe for diabetes patients.
- ***Nuts & seeds***: This includes items like cashews, pistachios, walnuts, sunflower seeds, pine nuts, flax seeds, almonds, and other nuts which may be your favorites. Keep these as a healthy snack throughout the day, but be sure to avoid the chocolate-covered or salted versions which are unhealthy. You would want to stick to the raw nuts. Chia seeds are also tiny but powerful! In just 2 tablespoons, you can have 11 grams of fiber! These are great to add to a smoothie or as a topping on oatmeal or cereal to fill you up. The great thing is that they are almost flavourless so anyone can incorporate them into their meals!
- ***Low-fat dairy***: If you are used to dairy products in your diet, you don't have to cut them out entirely but it's better to switch to low-fat versions. Make use fat-free yogurt or low-fat cheese and switch to skim or reduced fat milk. On the Mediterranean diet, you would want most of your dairy calories to come from healthy cheeses like feta, brie, Greek yogurt, or Parmesan.
- ***Herbs & spices:*** These are great to season your food with and they add a great distinct flavour other than salt. You can try using fresh herbs like rosemary and parsley,

though they may not last as long in your refrigerator. You can always start a windowsill herb garden which are easy to maintain! If not, don't be intimidated and feel free to use dried herbs from the spice aisle. Experiment with new flavours that will enhance your flavour profile. Fresh garlic and ginger are also great flavour enhancers and are considered essentials of Greek and Mediterranean cuisine. They have multiple health benefits and pack your meals with flavour.

Exclude:

- ***Red meat***: As we mentioned, you would want to go light on red meat portions when shopping for your Mediterranean diet. If you want to get a few portions, be sure they're smaller sized and lean meat cuts that have less fat. Try to only have it once a week and keep an eye on your portion size. Also, avoid high-fat processed meats like premade sausages or hot dogs that are loaded with preservatives and high in sodium. Ingesting them regularly will lead to inflammation in the body.
- ***Poultry***: Again, you would want to use poultry in your diet less often than you would on other diets. More lean cuts with less fat can be used now and then as long as you have smaller portions. For the most part, try and substitute your red meat and poultry meals with fish or seafood. However, it's okay to have them once in a while during the week. Turkey or duck would be a healthier alternative to chicken because they contain less fat.
- ***Refined grains***: These include things like bagels, cereal, or white bread that we might previously consider staples in our diet. But these should be excluded from your shopping list unless you have verified that the cereals, pasta, or bread are whole grain certified products.

- ***Sugars:*** This entails skipping things like candy, chocolate, ice cream, sugary juices, and sodas from your diet! Instead, try and treat yourself to berries or fruit as a sweet treat, or enhance your water with lemon or mint leaves for more flavour. Get used to the habit of having natural sugars in fruit as a dessert instead of wanting unhealthy baked goods.
- ***Trans or saturated fats***: Exclude things like butter or margarine which contain unhealthy saturated fats. You would want to substitute unhealthy oils like canola oil or vegetable oil with the healthier option of extra virgin olive oil. Also, you would want to use this in your cooking, frying, and as the main component of your vinaigrettes.
- ***Highly processed foods***: These should be avoided on the Mediterranean diet. The rule of thumb should be "if it comes in a box, you can't have it!" This is because food that tends to be marked as "low-fat" or "diet-friendly" is processed and unhealthy for your health. Instead of eating those empty calories, focus on what you can eat as a filling snack like some of the items we mentioned above.

SHOPPING GUIDE

Now that you have begun taking steps towards integrating the Mediterranean diet into your lifestyle, the time has come to go shopping. Stocking your refrigerator and pantry with the right ingredients will certainly go a long way in ensuring your success on this easy diet.

To make things easier for you and because I like to categorize, I have made a shopping list that will cover almost all your cooking needs:

Protein

- Unsalted nuts
- Fish and shellfish

- Beans, peas, and lentils
- Lean meats
- Skinless chicken and poultry where possible
- Poultry
- Eggs

Dairy

All dairy should either be low-fat or fat-free.

- Yogurt
- Sour cream
- Almond milk
- Rice milk
- Hemp milk
- Soy milk
- Cheese (try to find the low-fat cheeses)

Spices

- Salt
- Pepper
- Cinnamon
- Cumin
- Chili powder
- Cayenne pepper
- Curry powder
- Honey
- Vinegar
- Garlic
- Ginger
- Herbs

Whole grains

- Brown rice
- Quinoa

- Whole grain bread
- Whole wheat pasta
- Whole wheat flour, preferably stone milled
- Whole grain couscous

Vegetables

- Any fresh vegetables. Endeavor to incorporate a lot of dark leafy greens in your diet since they are full of antioxidants and other nutrients.
- Frozen vegetables.

Fruit

- Any fresh fruit that you enjoy. Aim to have seasonal fruits. This will help keep your budget cost-effective while you enjoy fresh produce.
- Frozen fruit

Pantry

- Seeds
- Oatmeal
- Chickpeas
- Black beans
- White beans
- Low-sodium broth

Other necessities

- Dry red wine such as cabernet sauvignon.
- Dark chocolate, roughly around the 70% mark.
- Unsweetened cocoa.

Whenever you see your kitchen running low on an item, write it down on a piece of paper on your fridge or your preferred method of keeping a shopping list. Top up your pantry every week and make sure you don't run short of any item. Every now and then, take a week or two to cook with the products you still have in your kitchen. This will help ensure that your food always stays relatively fresh and minimizes wastage.

Chapter Five
FUNDAMENTALS

Understanding the fundamentals surrounding the Mediterranean diet will empower and encourage you to stick with this healthy way of eating. There has been much controversy surrounding good fats vs. bad fats, red meat, and olive oil. In this chapter, I will bring some more clarity to these areas to help you understand how the Mediterranean diet functions, and how it will also benefit your health in the long-term. This is a mere introduction, but it should be fascinating nonetheless.

Good fats vs. bad fats – how do you choose?
When it comes to weight loss and health benefits, the fats you eat play a vital role. The dominant fat in your diet will either aggravate cardiovascular diseases, diabetes, cancer or obesity, or it will assist in regulating your moods, keep you mentally alert and regulate your weight.

How do you choose the fat that will give you benefits?
Knowing good fat from a bad one is the secret to a healthy life.

Saturated and trans fat fall under the **"bad fats"** category. Saturated fat is usually found in lard, fatty red meats, poultry skin, high fat dairy, and tropical oils such as coconut oil or palm oil. These saturated fats increase LDL (bad cholesterol), which is further aggravated when consumed with refined carbohydrates. Saturated fats increase the risk of cardiovascular diseases and type 2 diabetes.

Trans fats are even worse than saturated fats. They are found in margarine, fast foods, fried foods, vegetable shortening, processed snack foods, cookies, cakes, and pastries. These fats do not only raise LDL cholesterol, they also suppress HDL (good cholesterol), thereby elevating the risk of cardiovascular diseases three times higher than the risk involved in consuming saturated fats.

So what are the good fats?

So, good fats are monounsaturated fats and polyunsaturated fats. These fats can be found in natural products. Monounsaturated fats are found in nuts, avocados, vegetable oils, and olive oil.

Polyunsaturated fats are found in seafood, seeds and nuts. The best type of polyunsaturated fat is the omega-3 fatty acids found in salmon, sardines, trout, flaxseeds, or walnuts. Fish are is the best source for these fatty acids.

Another fantastic polyunsaturated fat is the omega-6 fatty acids found in tofu, walnuts, seeds, eggs, poultry, and so on.

These good fats improve blood cholesterol and reduce the risk of heart disease. Since fats generally has a high calorie content, moderation should still be used even when consuming good fats.

Let's look at olive oil extensively, since it is the Mediterranean diet's primary fat.

THE ROLE OF OLIVE OIL

Olive oil has many benefits that have flown under our radar. As the cornerstone of the Mediterranean diet, we must understand the role of olive oil plays in our health.

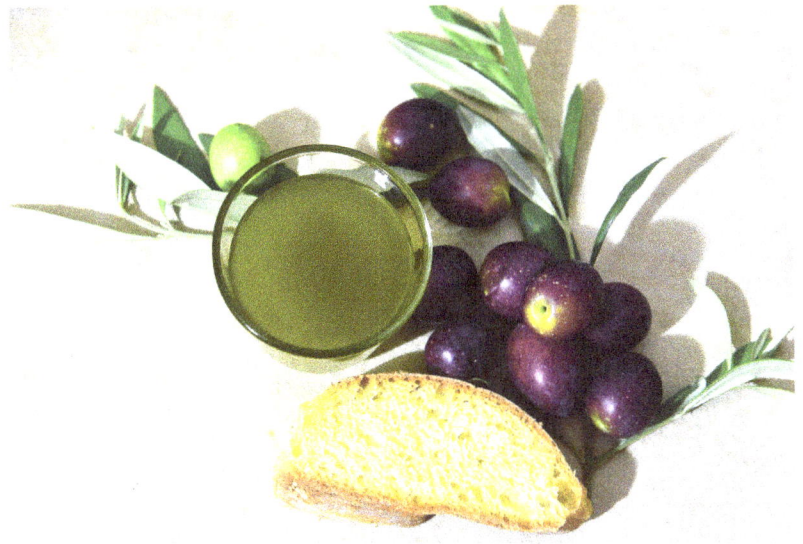

What is the best olive oil?

Olive oil is oil pressed from olives. The best olive oil is **extra virgin** olive oil or **EVOO,** which is naturally extracted and void of any solvents or cheaper oils. Make sure you purchase 100% natural **extra virgin** olive oil to give you the amazing health benefits.

Olive oil contains antioxidants that are known for their anti-inflammatory properties, including *oleocanthal*, an anti-inflammatory that works similar to ibuprofen in its anti-inflammatory effects, and *oleuropein*, which protects the body's LDL levels from oxidation. Olive oil also provides vitamins E and K.

Extra virgin olive oil has a higher amount of polyphenols and antioxidant agents that help with inflammation. They also reduce the effects of aging. These amazing polyphenols work with our microbiome to strengthen our immune system. When consumed with other foods rich in polyphenols, the impact on our health yields positive results. A **healthy gut** is key to a healthy body and polyphenols deals with that by enriching the digestive tract.

What are the other health benefits of olive oil?

. . .

Reduces risk of Type 2 Diabetes

Obesity and metabolic syndrome create a higher risk for developing Type 2 Diabetes. Studies show that a Mediterranean diet rich in olive oil improves blood sugar levels, insulin resistance and blood lipid levels. The result is the prevention of type 2 diabetes.

Potentially prevents strokes

Strokes occur when a blood clot blocks blood flow to the brain often causing brain damage or death to brain cells. **France has been conducting a study** that is part of the **Three-City Study** focused on the vascular risk factors for dementia. During their course of study, over 7,625 people (65 years and older) from three cities in France participated in this study. Some were given olive oil to use moderately in cooking while others were encouraged to use olive oil extensively.

After five years, researchers found that those who used olive oil in their diet had a 41% lower risk of strokes than those who did not incorporate olive oil in their diet.

Ensures a healthy heart

Olive oil protects the heart by doing the following:

- Protecting LDL cholesterol from oxidation.
- Improves the lining of blood vessels.
- Helps keep unwanted blood clots at bay.
- Reduces blood pressure.
- Reduces inflammation.

Fights osteoporosis

Osteoporosis occurs when bone mass decreases, thereby causing the bone tissues and bone to become fragile. People with osteoporosis are more susceptible to fractures at the slightest bump.

How we eat impacts the health of our bones. To keep the bones healthy, we must eat diets rich in calcium, vitamin D, phosphorus, magnesium, zinc, boron, iron, fluoride, copper. Recommended foods include nuts, seeds, beans, grains, fish, etc. Olive oil has been found to be a good source of calcium, iron, potassium, and sodium.

It is another reason to incorporate **extra virgin** olive oil in your diet.

Helps with cancer

Research has shown that olive oil assists in improving cell membrane function, which consequently lowers the risk of cancer. Olive oil also protects DNA from oxygen damage, thus helping our cells to function effectively. Research has also identified that oleocanthal helps prevent breast cancer cells from growing, while hydroxytyrosol kills colon cancer cells by helping the body block fatty acid synthetase (FAS) activity.

Another benefit of olive oil is its ability to protect the skin from the sun's UV rays. It also helps protect your cells against free radicals by neutralizing them.

In a nutshell, olive oil helps the body fight off cancer.

WINE AND BENEFITS

In the Mediterranean diet, wine is an enjoyable addition to a meal. Red wine is preferred over white wine for its heart benefits. Red wine seems to have a higher level of antioxidants than white wine. These antioxidants are a large contributor toward a healthy heart although it has not been concretely established.

Red wine contains flavonoids, which are high in antioxidants. Flavonoids are found in the grape skin. So if you can't have alcohol in your diet for various reasons, that's OK. You can still receive similar benefits by drinking red grape juice. Flavonoids lower LDL while increasing HDL. They also assist in reducing blood clotting. Flavonoids also help the body to resist allergens, viruses and carcinogens.

When it comes to choosing the red wine to go along with your meal, Merlots and red zinfandels may have more flavonoids than white wine, however, your dryer red wines are rich in flavonoid. Stock up on a few different brands of dry red wines to ensure that you get as many flavonoids and antioxidants as possible while enjoying your meal.

Other benefits that red wine seems to bring to its consumers include, assisting with weight loss, maintaining good memory, and controlling blood sugar. All thanks to resveratrol – a natural compound in grapes, peanuts, and mulberries, which is both antioxidant and anti-inflammatory.

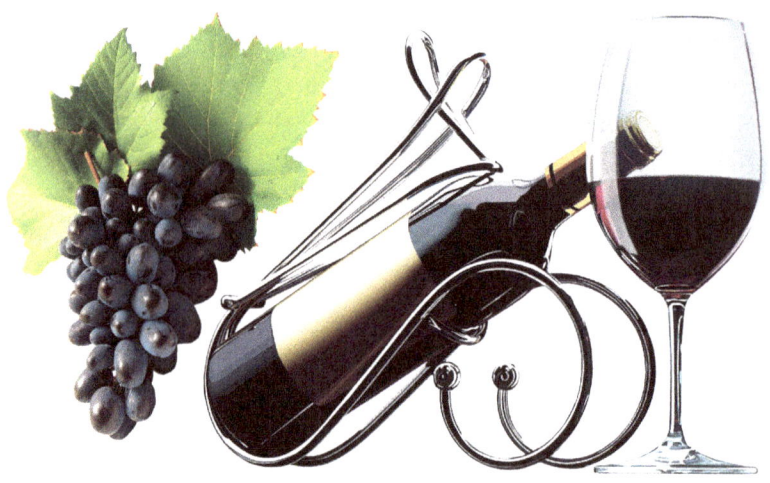

Wine yes...but with cautions

For red wine consumption to be healthy, you must stick to the recommended daily intake. Avoid alcohol if you have any of the following:

- Pancreatitis
- High blood pressure
- Liver disease
- Congestive heart failure.

When you have that delicious wine with your meal, savour your glass of wine, the food and your loved ones. Allow wine to enhance your meal and social experience. Remember, moderation is key for healthy living.

A WORD ON RED MEAT

Currently, there is a conflict which has led to the debate of red meat and its effect on the health of the heart. The Mediterranean diet traditionally tends to restrict red meat consumption to two servings per week, while white meat (poultry and fish) have a higher amount of weekly servings.

The current issue is not so much the red meat in general, but the processed red meats such as deli meats, bacon, and so on. Processed meat or any processed food is more detrimental to a person's health.

In this section, I am going to list some of the necessary nutrients that your body will receive when you consume lean unprocessed red meat (beef, pork, lamb). Lean red meats have been found to be fairly neutral with regards to their fatty acid profile, and as a result, their impact on cholesterol levels is more neutral than previously thought.

Lean red meats provide a variety of important micronutrients including the following:

- Zinc
- Iron
- Selenium
- Potassium
- B-vitamins
- Niacin
- Riboflavin
- Thiamine
- Vitamin B-12

All of these nutrients and more are essential to give your body the best health throughout your life. Particularly, children need a moderate supply of iron in their diets to assist their muscular development and amino blocks.

The link with red meat and cardiovascular disease lies in animal fat, which is saturated fat. Hence, consuming a fair portion of beef with fat trimmings may give you the essential micronutrients, but a lot of saturated fat at the same time. Here's my solution to this situation:

As you incorporate the Mediterranean diet into your lifestyle, look for lean cuts of beef. Buy extra lean mince, lean pork chops, and other lean meats such as veal. If you happen to buy red meat with fat on the edges, simply trim the fat off (either before or after cooking, depending on your purpose).

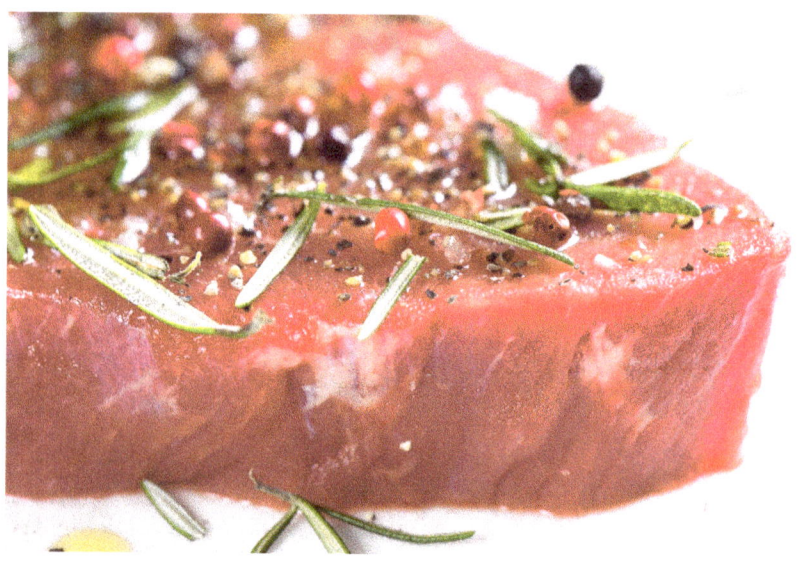

Chapter Six
ESSENTIAL NUTRIENTS & FOOD SOURCES

Each food contains different nutrients. In fact, a diet is well-balanced when you can get a good amount of fundamental nutrients from it. The Mediterranean diet is the most complete diet because it contains all kind of healthy foods.

Here's a list of nutrients you need to take each day and where you find them:

Protein - Proteins are macronutrients necessary for energy production, and it provides the body with materials necessary for growth. They are essential for the skin, hair, bones, they produce hormones, allow optimal functioning of the immune system. In the case of athletes, they are essential for muscle growth.

Carbohydrates - Carbohydrates are the first source of energy for our body and they include both simple sugars and complex carbohydrates. Our body can use carbohydrates instantly if it needs energy, or it can convert them into glycogen to store them as needed.

. . .

Fats – Fats, particularly phospholipids and cholesterol, are fundamental components of cell membranes. ... Our body needs at least 20g of fat daily to carry the fat-soluble vitamins.

Vitamins - Vitamins play an important role in the regulation of many chemical reactions that take place in our body and they are fundamental for a healthy life. They provide energy to the body and ensure cell renewal, guaranteeing protection for the skin, hair, teeth and preventing certain diseases.

Minerals - Unlike carbohydrates, proteins and fats, mineral (calcium, iron, zinc, etc) do not supply the body with energy, but are important in keeping it healthy. Their presence is fundamental for life-critical functions.

For example, some minerals are fundamental constituents of bones and teeth. Others are necessary for the functioning of enzymes, while others are fundamental for the functioning of some organs, such as iodine in the case of the thyroid.

NUTRIENTS FOOD SOURCES

- **Complex carbohydrate and fibre:** Pasta, wholemeal bread, wholegrain cereals, baked beans, peas, potatoes, other starchy vegetables.
- **Protein:** Lean meat, fish, chicken, eggs, milk, cheese, bread, nuts, legumes.
- **Fat:** Olive oil, nuts.
- **Vitamin A:** Eggs, cheese, meat.
- **Beta-carotene*(converts to vitamin A)*:** Carrots, pumpkin, spinach, tomatoes, broccoli, apricots, rockmelon.
- **Vitamin D:** Eggs, cheese.
- **Vitamin E:** Olive oil, nuts, fatty fish, a small percentage also in green vegetables and wholegrain cereals.

- **Vitamin K:** Eggs, pork, cheese, green vegetables.
- **Thiamin:** Wholegrain cereals, pork, bread, peas, nuts.
- **Riboflavin:** Meat, milk, eggs, wholegrain, cheese, cereals, mushrooms, nuts.
- **Niacin:** Fish, meat, wholegrain cereals, mushrooms, peanuts, nuts.
- **Pantothenic acid:** Wholegrain cereals, eggs, meat, fish, peanuts, vegetables.
- **Vitamin B6:** Meat, fish, wholegrain cereals, bananas, peanuts.
- **Folic acid:** Green vegetables, wholegrain cereals, nuts.
- **Vitamin B12:** Eggs, meat, fish, milk, oysters.
- **Biotin:** Milk, cheese, fish, eggs, wholegrain cereals.
- **Vitamin C:** Oranges, strawberries, tomatoes, broccoli, cabbage, potatoes, Brussels sprouts.
- **Calcium:** Milk, cheese, yoghurt, nuts, sesame seeds.
- **Phosphorus:** Fish, poultry, meat, eggs, milk, cheese, nuts, bread, cereals.
- **Iron:** Meat, poultry, eggs, wholemeal bread, wholegrain cereals.
- **Sodium:** Seafood, meat, spinach, celery, milk, cheese.
- **Potassium:** Bananas, potatoes, apricots, oranges, fish, meat, nuts.
- **Iodine:** Sea foods, milk, cereals, vegetables (preferably from areas with high iodine content in the soil)
- **Zinc:** Oysters, fish, meat, poultry, eggs, peanuts, wholegrain cereals.

Chapter Seven
GETTING STARTED

Now that we have dissected the Mediterranean diet, let's put it all back together and see how we can move from our current eating habits to a Mediterranean lifestyle. In this chapter, you will find the right information on how to integrate the Mediterranean diet into your life, what to add to your shopping list, tips for eating out, and ideal portion sizes.

MOVING TO THE MEDITERRANEAN DIET

In Chapter 3, I listed the daily and weekly portions of food when I elaborated on the Mediterranean diet pyramid. Following this pyramid will help you transition into the Mediterranean diet. Below are a few more tips to help you transition:

- Incorporate more fruits and vegetables into your diet by adding them to your meals and using them as snacks.
- Replace refined bread and pasta with whole grains.
- Increase your fish intake while reducing your red meat.
- Change your dairy from high fat to low fat or skim milk.

- Sauté food in olive oil. Olive oil is your dominant fat – try to use it for everything you cook.
- Eat slowly. The slower you eat the more time you give your body to register that it has food to process in your stomach. This will also reduce acid reflux and indigestion.
- Clean out the kitchen of unhealthy foods. The reality is, we eat whatever is in the fridge or pantry. Remove temptation by giving your unhealthy foods away to shelters in your kitchen or storeroom or consume them before moving on to the Mediterranean diet.
- Start small. Notice what you normally eat and gradually replace it with a healthier option. This can be a gentler way of transitioning your body and mind towards a healthy diet. As the saying goes, **Rome wasn't built in a day**. Take it one step at a time.
- Reduce your salt intake where possible. Salt is known to encourage water retention amongst other things. Cook with salt and avoid adding salt to your food after its cooked

FOOD TO EAT

Fruits and vegetables

Mediterranean diet is one of the plant-based diet plans. Fresh fruits and vegetables contain a large number of vitamins, nutrients, fibers, minerals, and antioxidants.

Fruits: Apple, berries, grapes, peaches, fig, grapefruit, dates, melon, oranges and pears.

Vegetables: Spinach, Brussels sprout, kale, tomatoes, kale, summer squash, onion, cauliflower, peppers, cucumbers, turnips, potatoes, sweet potatoes, and parsnips.

Seeds and nuts

Seeds and nuts are rich in monounsaturated fats and omega-3 fatty acids.

Seeds: Pumpkin seeds, flax seeds, sesame seeds, and sunflower seeds.

Nuts: Almond, hazelnuts, pistachios, cashews, and walnuts.

WHOLE GRAINS

Whole grains are high in fibers, and they are not processed so they do not contain unhealthy fats like trans-fats compared to processed ones.

Whole grains: Wheat, quinoa, rice, barley, oats, rye, and brown rice. You can also use bread and pasta which is also made from whole grains.

OILY FISH AND SEAFOOD

Fish are the rich source of omega-3 fatty acids and proteins. Eating fish at least once a week is recommended here. The healthiest way to consume fish is to grill it. Grilling fish taste good and it doesn't need extra oil.

Fish and seafood: Salmon, trout, clams, mackerel, sardines, tuna and shrimp.

LEGUMES

Legumes (beans) are a rich source of protein, vitamins, and fibers. Regular consumption of beans helps to reduce the risk of diabetes, cancer and heart disease.

Legumes: Kidney beans, peas, chickpeas, black beans, fava beans, lentils, and pinto beans.

SPICES AND HERBS

Spices and herbs are used to add taste to meals.

Spices and herbs: Mint, thyme, garlic, basil, cinnamon, nutmeg, rosemary, oregano and more.

. . .

Healthy fats

Olive oil is the main fat used in the Mediterranean diet. It helps to reduce the risk of inflammatory disorder, diabetes, cancer, and heart-related disease. It also helps to increase HDL (good cholesterol) levels and decrease LDL (bad cholesterol) levels in the body. It also helps in weight reduction.

Fats: Olive oil, avocado oil, walnut oil, extra virgin olive oil, avocado, and olives.

Dairy

Moderate amounts of dairy products are utilized in the Mediterranean diet. The dairy product contains high amounts of fats.

Dairy: Greek yogurt, skim milk and cheese.

FOOD TO AVOID

Refined grains

Refined grains like white bread, white rice, and pasta are not allowed or utilized in a Mediterranean diet. They raise your blood sugar level.

Refined oils

Oils like canola oils, cottonseed oils, and soybean oils are completely avoided in a Mediterranean diet. This is because they raise your LDL (bad cholesterol) level.

Added Sugar

These types of artificial sugars are found in table sugar, soda, chocolate, ice cream, and candies. They raise your blood sugar level.

TIPS: You should consume only natural sugars in the Mediterranean diet.

. . .

PROCESSED FOODS

Generally, processed foods come in boxes as well as any items labeled "diet" or "low-fat". They contain a high amount of trans-fats.

TIPS: Mediterranean diet is all about eating fresh and natural food.

TRANS-FAT AND SATURATED FATS

In this category, food contains butter and margarine.

PROCESSED MEAT

Typical processed meat such as bacon, hot dogs and sausage.

8 TIPS FOR SUCCESS

Here are some simple but effective guidelines to start a Mediterranean diet in no time! These tips are based on the traditional Greek and Italian diet, from which the authentic Mediterranean diet was based. They include;

1. **Never skip breakfast** - Breakfast remains the most important meal of the day for a large number of experts among nutritionists and dieticians. Luckily, fewer people are applying the old belief of skipping breakfast to lose weight easily. Paradoxically, not eating in the morning can make you gain more weight because it slows down the body's metabolism.
2. **Change your lifestyle** - Share food with family and friends by celebrating valuable moments and going for a walk together. Union makes the force and it will help you keep on the right path in following the Mediterranean lifestyle.
3. **Add whole grain and brown rice** - Mediterranean diet recommends brown rice and whole grains in the diet because grains are the best source of protein and they are

rich in fibers. The bowl of oatmeal is one of the perfect breakfasts during the cold season.

4. **Shop locally and seasonal** - Shopping locally ensures that you get the freshest product possible. Fruit and vegetables that follow their normal life cycle have a greater amount of nutrients and provide the right amount of calories in relation to the time of year. Seasonal products are better, fragrant, aromatic and also cost less, given the lower cost for production.
5. **Keep fruit and seeds ready**- Fruits and seeds are an essential part of the Mediterranean diet. Keep a jar of mixed nuts on your kitchen counter and eat a handful of those along with your vegetable or fruit snack..
6. **Manage portions, not calories** - Always keep an eye on your portions, and don't concentrate on counting calories. Instead, try to manage the quality of calories in your portions. As I previously explained, rearrange your dishes for the type of calories you will ingest.
7. **Serving fruit as dessert instead of sweet** - Fruit can be used as desserts or as snacks. You can also prepare delicious desserts using fruit and replacing all parts of the butter with olive oil.
8. **Focus on the meal** - While eating your meal, you must concentrate on your meat. Always eat your meal slowly and give yourself 20 minutes to eat a meal. Stop eating your food in front of the television. You must focus and concentrate on your meal while eating.

TIPS TO EATING OUT

Going out for dinner is permitted on most diets and the Mediterranean diet is no different. Making wise choices while out at a restaurant for dinner can go a long way to help you keep a healthy momentum.

. . .

Share an appetizer

An appetizer is meant to be a palette tickler. It should be a little bit of food to take the hunger pains away while setting the tone for the remainder of the evening. Order an appetizer that can be shared between you and two other people, or order a small platter for the whole table (depending on the size of your table).

Share your main meal

If you and a friend or your partner are ordering the same food, why not share a plate? Sharing a plate of food will regulate the portion size to fit more within the recommended size. Most restaurants tend to provide large plates of food that can easily be split into two meals.

If you don't have someone to share your food with, eat half and request for the remaining half to be placed in a take away for your next meal.

Say no to fried food

Where you have the option to replace fried food (chips or onion rings) with steamed, raw, or grilled vegetables, seize the opportunity and do so. Request for rice or baked potato instead of chips.

Request for your food to be grilled not fried where possible. You can also make a specific request for your food to be cooked in olive oil and not unhealthy fats.

Choose your drink

Have a cappuccino, tea, seltzer water, glass of wine, or diet soda while eating out.

Dessert

If you want dessert, request for fresh fruits. If you can't come up with a more "healthy" dessert, share a dessert with the table or hold off until you get home.

Chapter Eight
HOW TO MANAGE PORTIONS?

If you ask me "what's the #1 suggestion to actually eat in a healthy way?" I will surely suggest you follow the food scheme of the Mediterranean diet pyramid. This is a scheme that provides a balanced number of portions to eat different types of food. Thanks to this scheme you will obtain a nutritional balance that corresponds correctly to the Mediterranean diet philosophy.

The pyramid has at its base the foods to consume in each main meal (fruit, vegetables and cereals), then those to eat daily (oil, dairy products, nuts) and those to eat only a few times a week (meat, fish, legumes, desserts).

Now, I know that I have to eat at least 5 portions of fruit and vegetables a day. But, how much is a portion? And the same goes for other foods; how much is a portion of meat or pasta or dairy products?

The answer comes from IOM, the Institute Of Medicine of the National Academies (United States), which through the work of dozens of scientists and experts updated in 2016, the so-called DRI (Dietary Reference Intake), has set of values used to plan and assess nutrient intake of healthy people.

Thus, leafing through the indications that come from IOM, it turns out the following correct portions:

- Milk and yogurt - 125 grams.
- Fresh cheeses - 100 grams, while mature cheeses - 50 grams.
- The correct portion for meat - 100 grams, while cured meats - 50 grams
- Fish and seafood - 150 grams
- Eggs - 50 grams
- Fresh legumes - 150 grams, which become 50 for dry ones
- Cereals - 50 grams for bread, while for pasta, rice, spelled and barley the portion is 80 grams.
- Salad - 80 grams.
- Vegetables (raw and cooked) - 200 grams
- Fruit - 150 grams

It is clear that the calories needed, the number of portions, or the quantities to eat vary quite significantly in children, an elderly person, both man and woman. Just as the weight, lifestyle and amount of physical activities must be taken into consideration.

So to establish the correct nutrition of a person, the general schemes and information on the correct portions are certainly useful, but it is also necessary to modulate them taking into series of elements and factors that only that person knows and on which, in case of doubts, is good to consult doctors and nutritionists, wary of the DIY that often ramps.

Portion sizes

Personally, I have often struggled to get the right portion sizes for each meal. At times, I wondered if the recommended portion sizes are too small or too big. Knowing the practical ways to regulate portion sizes goes a long way to removing this ambiguity.

- One serving of fresh fruit = ½ cup
- One serving of raw vegetables = 1 cup
- One serving of cooked vegetables = ½ cup
- One serving of protein = the size of your palm (the base of your fingers to the wrist).

- One serving of bread = 1 slice
- One serving of cooked pasta or brown rice = ½ cup

Now, time to get cooking!

Part One

BREAKFAST

BREAKFAST QUESADILLA

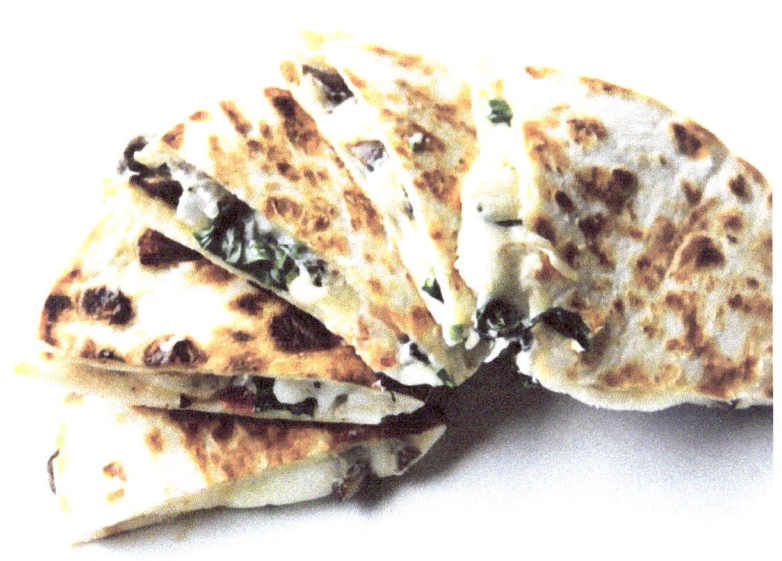

PREPARATION TIME: 5 MINUTES

Cooking time: 10 minutes
Servings: 2

Ingredients:

- 1 Skinless Boneless Chicken Breast
- 2 Large Eggs
- 2 Egg Whites
- 1 cup of Chopped Baby Spinach
- 1 tablespoon of Extra-Virgin Olive Oil
- 1/2 cup of Chopped Tomatoes
- 1/4 cup of Sour Cream
- 2/3 cup of Shredded Cheddar and Jack Cheese Blend
- 1 Pitted and Chopped Avocado
- 1/4 cup of Sliced Black Olives
- 3 Sliced Green Onions
- 2 tablespoons of Chopped Fresh Cilantro
- Salsa
- Tortillas

Directions:
Chicken:

1. Preheat your broiler.
2. Pound your chicken breast lightly using a meat pounder.
3. Season with pepper and salt. Broil on your broiler pan for approximately 4 to 5 minutes on each side. Cook until the chicken is done and no longer pink on the inside.
4. Transfer to your chopping board and dice the chicken breast.

Quesadilla:

1. Preheat your oven to 200 degrees.
2. In a bowl, whisk your eggs together.

3. Heat your oil in a frying pan over a medium heat.
4. Add your egg mixture to your pan and cook until the edges have begun to set.
5. Stir with your spatula, scraping eggs on the bottom and sides of your pan and fold them toward the center.
6. Add your spinach, chicken, and tomatoes. Continue to cook.
7. Stir frequently until your eggs are fluffy and light. Remove your pan from heat and set to the side.
8. Drizzle olive oil on a separate frying pan over a medium heat. Place a tortilla in a pan and heat up until it is warmed.
9. Flip your tortilla and sprinkle the bottom half with 1/3 cup of your cheese mixture.
10. Top your cheese with half of your egg mixture.
11. Fold your tortilla in half in your pan to cover the eggs and cheese.
12. Cook until golden brown on the bottom of tortilla.
13. Flip your quesadilla and cook the opposite side until golden brown.
14. Transfer to your baking sheet to keep it warm while cooking your second quesadilla.
15. Cut each into wedges. Top with cilantro, sour cream, avocado, olives, green onions, and salsa.

Nutrition Values: calories 230, fat 12g, fiber 12g, carbs 34g, protein 13g

HEARTY BREAKFAST FRITTATA W/ TOMATO SALAD

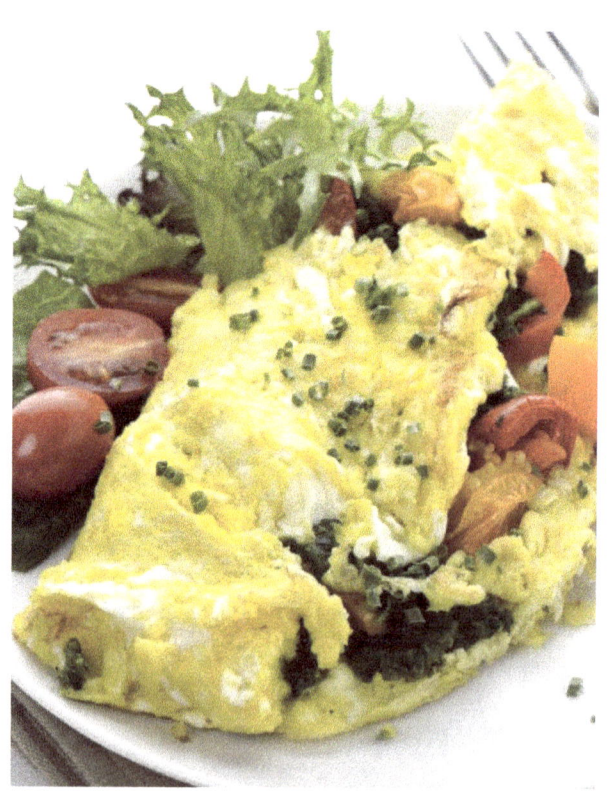

Preparation time: 5 minutes
Cooking time: 27 minutes
Servings: 4

Ingredients:

- 4 Eggs
- 1 tablespoon of Vegetable Oil
- 1 2/3 pounds of Sliced and Peeled Potatoes
- 2 Onions (1 Diced / 1 Sliced Into Rings)
- 1 Small Diced Zucchini
- 1 ounce of Pitted and Sliced Black Olives
- 5 1/4 ounces of Diced Salami
- 12 ounces of Diced Tomatoes
- 1/3 cup of Whipping Cream
- 5 sprigs of Sliced Basil
- 1 teaspoon of Balsamic Vinegar
- 2 tablespoons of Olive Oil

Directions:

1. Heat your vegetable oil in a pan and fry your potatoes for approximately 12 minutes.
2. Add your onion rings, zucchini, olives, and salami. Saute for another 5 minutes.
3. Beat your cream and eggs together. Season them and pour over the vegetables. Cover and cook over a medium heat for approximately 10 minutes.
4. Toss together your diced onions, diced tomatoes, vinegar, olive oil, and basil. Season to taste. Slice your frittata into quarters and arrange with your tomato salad on plates.
5. Serve and Enjoy!

Nutrition Values: calories 250, fat 12g, fiber 12g, carbs 34g, protein 13g

SPAGHETTI FRITTATA

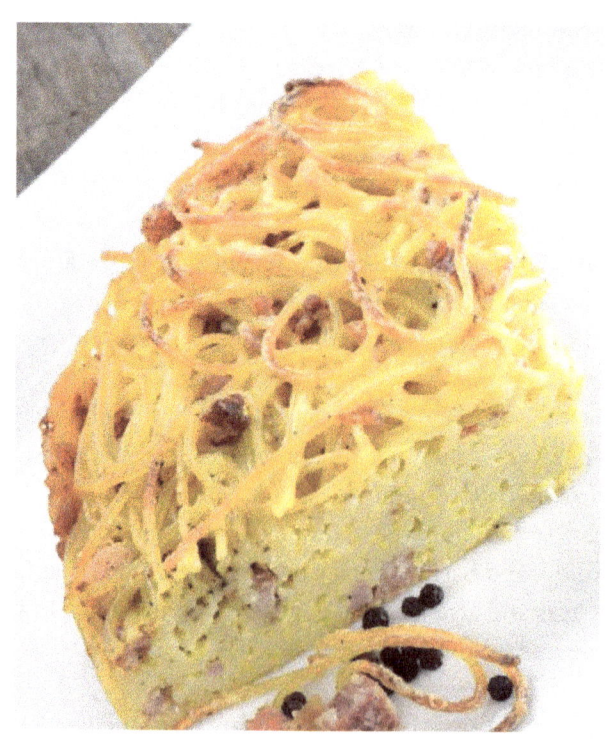

PREPARATION TIME: 5 MINUTES
COOKING TIME: 30 MINUTES
SERVINGS: 6

Ingredients:

- 6 Large Eggs
- 2 cups of Cooked Spaghetti
- 4 slices of Bacon
- 2 cloves of Minced Garlic
- 1 Diced Purple Onion
- 1 cup of Grated Mozzarella Cheese
- 1/4 cup of Grated Parmesan Cheese
- 3 ounces of Chopped Spinach
- 2 cloves of Minced Garlic
- 1/4 cup of Sliced Black Olives
- 6 Grape Tomatoes
- 1 tablespoon of Fresh Basil Leaves
- Ground Black Pepper
- Salt

Directions:

1. In a big bowl, whisk your parmesan cheese and eggs until well blended. Season with pepper and salt. Add your spaghetti and toss it so everything gets combined. Set aside.
2. Preheat your oven to 375 degrees. In a large cast iron skillet over a medium heat, cook your bacon until it is crisp and set on paper towels to drain. Add onion to your skillet and saute over a medium heat approximately 5 minutes. Stir it often until softened. Add your spinach and cook it until it has wilted. Should take 2 minutes. Add your garlic and saute until it becomes fragrant. Should take about 1 minute.
3. Pour your spaghetti egg mixture into your skillet and sprinkle with your bacon pieces. Add your mozzarella,

tomatoes, basil, and olives on top. Lower your heat and allow to cook for 3 minutes until the eggs have set on the bottom. Transfer your pan into the oven and cook for approximately 15 to 20 minutes. Remove from the oven and let it cool before serving.
4. Serve and Enjoy!

Nutrition Values: calories 274, fat 11.6g, fiber 2.8g, carbs 13.5g, protein 15.4g

CHICKPEA & POTATO HASH

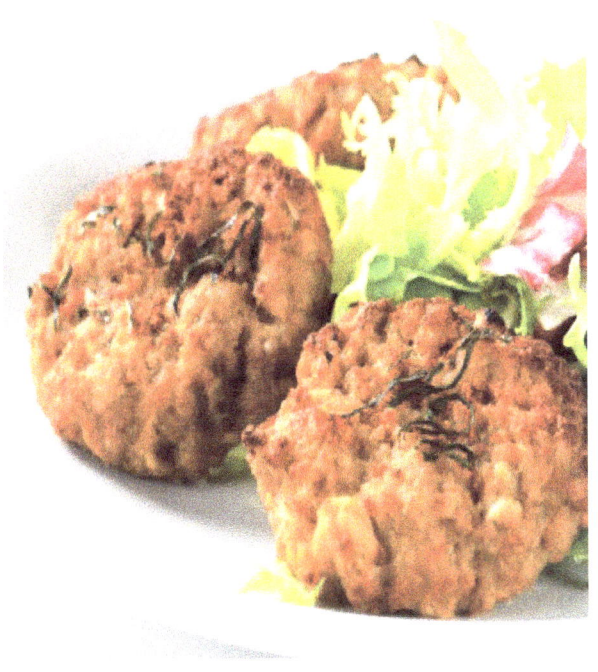

PREPARATION TIME: 5 MINUTES
COOKING TIME: 10 MINUTES
SERVINGS: 4

Ingredients:

- 4 cups of Frozen Shredded Hash Brown Potatoes
- 1/2 cup of Finely Chopped Onion
- 2 cups of Finely Chopped Baby Spinach
- 1 tablespoon of Minced Fresh Ginger
- 1/2 teaspoon of Salt
- 1 tablespoon of Curry Powder
- 1/4 cup of Extra-Virgin Olive Oil
- 4 Large Eggs
- 1 (15-ounce) can of Chickpeas
- 1 cup of Chopped Zucchini

Directions:

1. Combine your spinach, potatoes, ginger, onion, salt, and curry powder in a big bowl. Heat your oil in a large sized skillet over a medium-high heat. Add in your potato mixture and press down into a layer. Cook mixture without stirring. Cook until golden brown on bottom and crispy. Should take approximately 3 to 5 minutes.
2. Reduce the heat to a medium-low. Fold in your zucchini and chickpeas. Once folded in, press your mixture back into an even layer. Carve 4 wells out in your mixture. Break your eggs, one at a time and slip into each of your wells. Cover and continue to cook until your eggs are set. Should take approximately 4 to 5 minutes.
3. Serve and Enjoy!

Nutrition Values: calories 400, fat 32g, fiber 0g, carbs 2g, protein 24g

MEDITERRANEAN BREAKFAST QUINOA

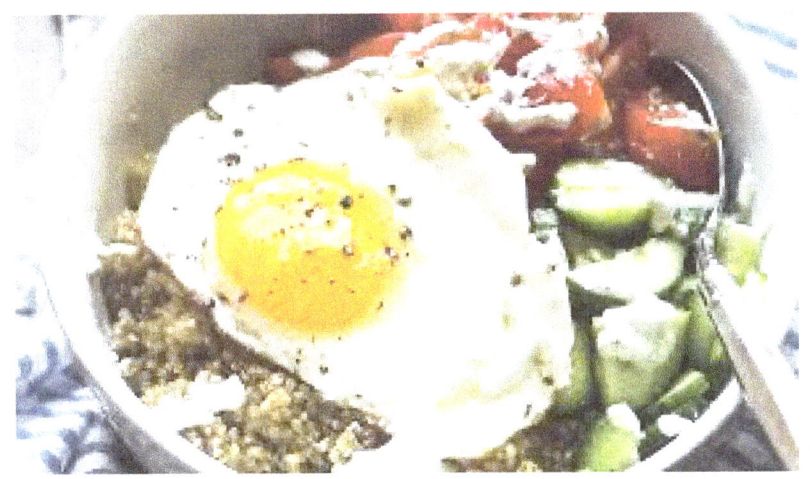

Preparation time: 5 minutes
Cooking time: 20 minutes
Servings: 4

Ingredients:

- 1 teaspoon of Ground Cinnamon
- 1/4 cup of Chopped Raw Almonds
- 2 cups of Milk
- 1 cup of Quinoa
- 1 teaspoon of Vanilla Extract
- 1 teaspoon of Sea Salt
- 2 Chopped Dried Pitted Dates
- 2 tablespoons of Honey
- 5 Chopped Dried Apricots

Directions:

1. Toast your almonds in your skillet over a medium heat. Should take approximately 3 to 5 minutes until golden. Set them aside.
2. Heat your quinoa and cinnamon together in your saucepan over a medium heat.
3. Add the sea salt and milk to your saucepan. Stir in well.
4. Bring your mixture to a boil, reduce the heat to low. Cover your saucepan and allow to simmer for approximately 15 minutes.
5. Stir in your honey, dates, vanilla, apricots, and 1/2 of your toasted almonds.
6. Pour rest of almonds on top when ready to serve.
7. Serve and Enjoy!

Nutrition Values: calories 500, fat 28g, fiber 4g, carbs 12g, protein 56g

BREAKFAST ENCHILADAS

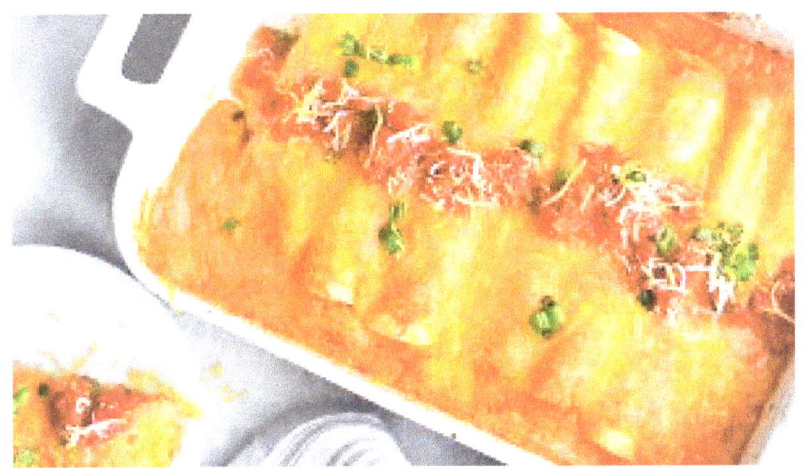

Preparation time: 5 minutes
Cooking time: 1 hour & 15 minutes
Servings: 4

. . .

Ingredients:

- 14 Large Eggs
- 8 ounces of Spicy Vegetarian Breakfast Sausages
- 2 tablespoons of Butter
- 4 Sliced Green Onions
- 2 tablespoons of Chopped Fresh Cilantro
- 1/2 teaspoon of Pepper
- 3/4 teaspoon of Salt
- 8 Whole Wheat Tortillas
- 1 cup of Shredded Pepper Jack Cheese
- 1/3 cup of Flour
- 3 cups of Milk
- 1/3 cup of Butter
- 2 cups of Shredded Cheddar Cheese
- 4 1/2 ounces of Chopped Green Chiles
- 1/2 cup of Grape Tomatoes
- 1/8 cup of Sliced Black Olives

Directions:

1. Melt the butter in a saucepan over a medium heat. Whisk in the flour until it is smooth. Cook, constantly whisking for approximately 1 minute. Gradually, whisk in your milk and continue to cook over a medium heat. Whisk constantly until mixture has thickened. Should take approximately 5 minutes. Remove from heat. Whisk in your green chiles, cheddar cheese, and salt.
2. Cook your sausage. Remove from pan when finished. Drain if necessary.
3. Melt butter in a large skillet over a medium heat. Add in your cilantro and green onions. Saute them. Add your salt, eggs, and pepper. Cook without any stirring until your eggs have begun to set. Bring your spatula across the bottom of your pan to help distribute uncooked eggs. Keep cooking until the eggs have gotten thick but are still moist. Remove

from the heat and fold in your sausage and 1 1/2 cups of cheese sauce from the first step.
4. Spoon 1/3 of a cup of your egg mixture down the center of each of your tortillas and roll up. Place the seam side down in a greased 13 x 9 baking dish. Repeat for all your tortillas. Pour your remaining cheese mixture over the tortillas evenly and sprinkle with pepper jack cheese. Refrigerate approximately 45 minutes.
5. Bake at 350 degrees for approximately 30 minutes or until your cheese is bubbling. Sprinkle with the toppings of your choice.
6. Serve and Enjoy!

Nutrition Values: calories 340, fat 3g, fiber 4g, carbs 12g, protein 20g

MEDITERRANEAN BREAKFAST WRAPS

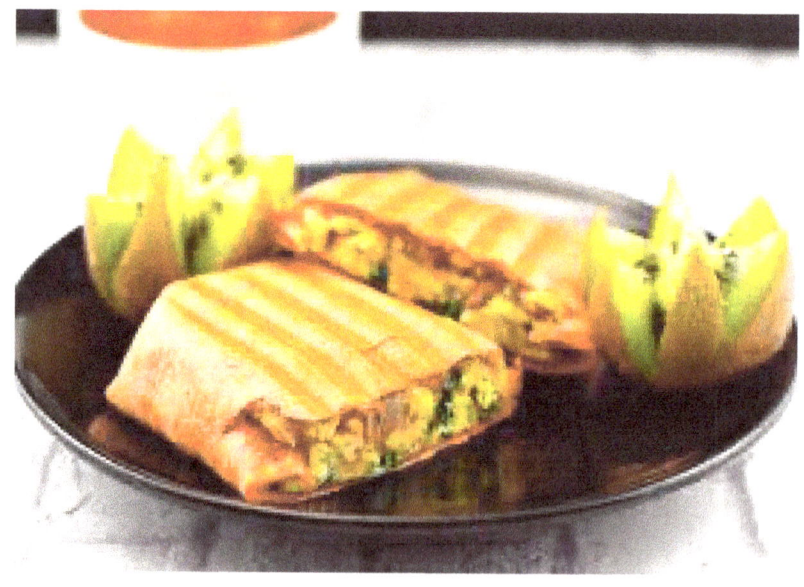

Preparation time: 5 minutes
Cooking time: 15 minutes

Servings: 4

Ingredients:

- 4 Eggs
- 4 Tortillas
- 1 tablespoon of Water
- 1/2 teaspoon of Garlic Chipotle Seasoning
- 4 tablespoons of Crumbled Feta Cheese
- 4 tablespoons of Tomato Chutney
- 1 cup of Chopped Fresh Spinach Leaves
- Dried Tomatoes
- Bacon
- Prosciutto
- Salt
- Pepper

Directions:

1. Mix your eggs, seasoning, and water.
2. Heat a skillet. Add some butter or bacon grease. Add in your egg mixture and scramble for 3 to 4 minutes until cooked.
3. Lay your tortillas out and divide your eggs among them evenly. Leave the edges free so you can fold them.
4. Top each layer of your eggs with an even amount of cheese. Approximately 1 tablespoon for each wrap.
5. Add tomato chutney. Approximately 1 tablespoon for each wrap.
6. Add spinach. Approximately 1/4 cup for each wrap.
7. Add bacon and prosciutto. I use a couple of slices on each wrap but feel free to add the amount you prefer.
8. Roll up the tortillas burrito style. Be sure to fold in both of your ends.

9. Cook approximately 1 minute on a skillet or panini maker.
10. Serve and Enjoy!

Nutrition Values: calories 340, fat 3g, fiber 4g, carbs 12g, protein 20g

PANERA MEDITERRANEAN BREAKFAST SANDWICH

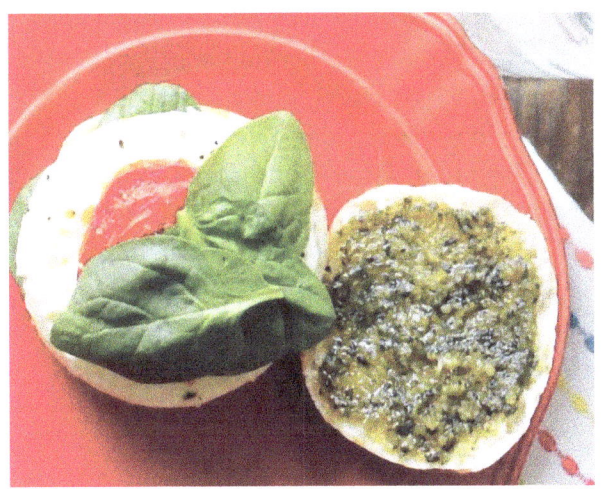

Preparation time: 5 minutes
Cooking time: 2 minutes
Servings: 1

. . .

Ingredients:

- 2 Egg Whites
- 1 Ciabatta Roll
- 1 slice of Tomato
- 1 slice of White Cheddar Cheese
- 1 tablespoon of Pesto
- 1 handful of Baby Spinach
- Cracked Black Pepper

Directions:

1. Split your roll and place the cheese on bottom half.
2. Lightly broil the half of roll with cheese on it in your toaster oven.
3. Spray a ramekin or mug with cooking spray. Pour eggs whites into it and cover. Microwave for approximately 45 to 60 seconds. Place tomato slice on top of your cooked egg and microwave it for about 10 more seconds.
4. Place your cooked egg and tomato on top of your cheese covered half of roll. Sprinkle the top with cracked pepper. Spread pesto on the top half of your roll. Add spinach on top of the tomato and put your sandwich together.
5. Serve and Enjoy!

Nutrition Values: calories 274, fat 11.6g, fiber 2.8g, carbs 13.5g, protein 15.4g

GREEK SCRAMBLE

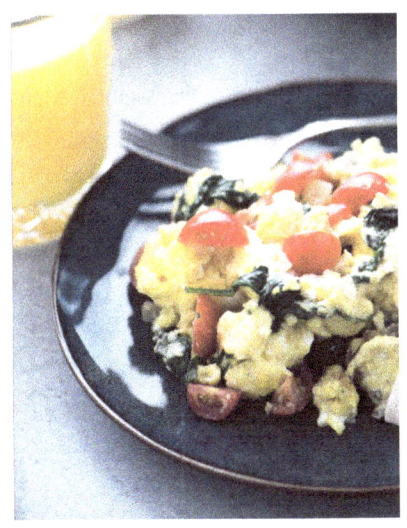

Preparation time: 5 minutes
Cooking time: 15 minutes
Servings: 4

. . .

Ingredients:

- 10 Large Eggs
- 1/4 cup of Milk
- 2/3 cup of Crumbled Feta Cheese
- 1/2 teaspoon of Fine Salt
- 1 tablespoon of Olive Oil
- 1/4 teaspoon of Ground Black Pepper
- 6 ounces of Baby Spinach
- 1/2 Diced Yellow Onion
- 1 cup of Quartered Cherry Tomatoes
- Pita Bread

Directions:

1. Whisk your eggs, salt, pepper, and milk in a large bowl. Set to the side.
2. Heat your oil in a skillet over a medium heat until simmering. Add your onion. Stir occasionally, cook approximately 5 minutes. Add the spinach, tossing until completely wilted and no liquid is left. Should take approximately 3 minutes.
3. Reduce your heat to a medium-low and pour in your egg mixture. Cook for 2 minutes. Using a rubber spatula, push your set eggs from the edge of the skillet to the center. Spread your uncooked eggs back into an even layer. Repeat, pushing the set eggs from edges to the center every 30 seconds until they are all nearly set. Total cooking time should be approximately 6 minutes.
4. Remove skillet from the heat and fold in your tomatoes. Toast your pita bread.
5. Serve and Enjoy!

Nutrition Values: Calories 202, Protein 2.5g, Carbs 25.5g, Fat 10g

CHEESY MEDITERRANEAN SCRAMBLE

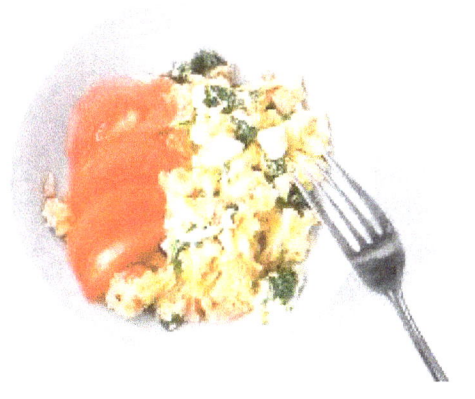

Preparation time: 5 minutes
Cooking time: 10 minutes
Servings: 6

. . .

Ingredients:

- 6 slices of Whole Wheat Bread
- 3 cartons of Egg Substitute
- 1/8 teaspoon of Ground Black Pepper
- 1/2 teaspoon of Crushed Dried Basil Leaves
- 1 1/2 tablespoons of Butter Spread
- 2 tablespoons of Low Fat Feta Cheese
- 1 Small Chopped Red Pepper
- 1 Small Chopped Sweet Onion

Directions:

1. In a large bowl add egg substitute, black pepper, and basil. Whisk and set aside.
2. In a 10-inch skillet, melt your butter spread over a medium-high heat and cook your onion and red pepper. Stir occasionally for 4 minutes until the vegetables get tender. Stir in your egg mixture and allow it to set slightly.
3. Cook eggs until set, stirring occasionally. Sprinkle with cheese. Toast your slices of white bread.
4. Serve and Enjoy!

Nutrition Values: calories 340, fat 3g, fiber 4g, carbs 12g, protein 20g

MEDITERRANEAN OMELET

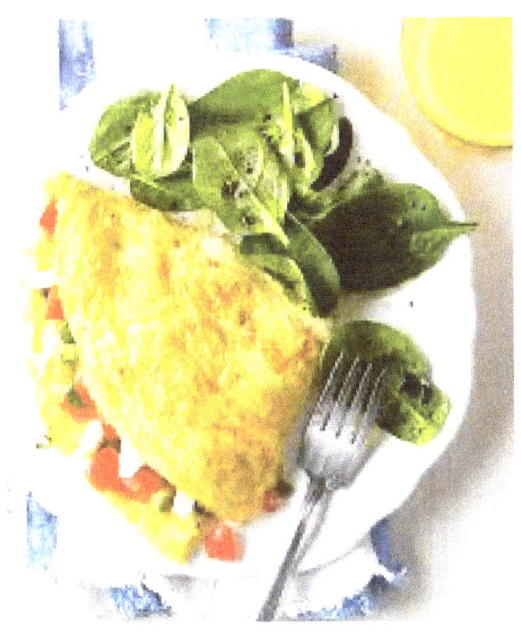

Preparation time: 5 minutes
Cooking time: 10 minutes

Servings: 4

Ingredients:

- 2 Large Eggs
- 1 Tomato
- 1 teaspoon of Olive Oil
- 3 sprigs of Chives
- 4 1/4 tablespoons of Feta Cheese
- 1/2 teaspoon of Dried Oregano
- Olives
- Pinch of Salt

Directions:

1. In frying pan heat your olive oil.
2. Add your chopped tomato, oregano, and onion. Cook until the tomatoes are no longer soft.
3. Add in your olives and turn the heat off. Add your feta cheese.
4. In a different frying pan add your eggs and salt and cook.
5. Combine ingredients and add your toppings.
6. Serve and Enjoy!

Nutrition Values: calories 250, fat 13.9g, fiber 11.1g, carbs 23.8g, protein 17.5g

HUEVOS REVUELTOS

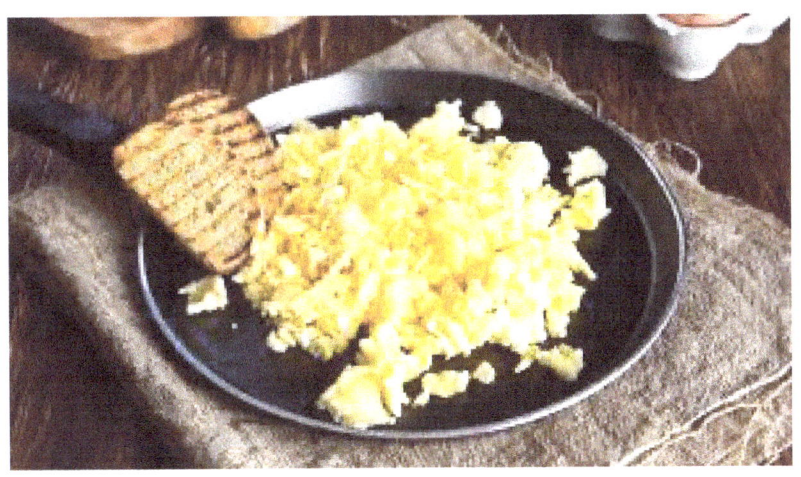

Preparation time: 5 minutes
Cooking time: 6 minutes
Servings: 4

. . .

Ingredients:

- 4 Eggs
- 2 tablespoons of Butter Spread
- 1/4 cup of Crumbled Queso Fresco Cheese
- 1/2 cup of Chopped Tomatoes
- 1/2 cup of Chopped Onion
- Chopped Fresh Cilantro

Directions:

1. Melt your butter spread in a skillet over a medium heat and add your vegetables. Stir occasionally, approximately 4 minutes or until they are tender. Add in your eggs. Stir frequently, approximately 2 minutes until the eggs are done.
2. Sprinkle with your cilantro and cheese.
3. Serve and Enjoy!

Nutrition Values: Calories 202; Protein 2.5g, Carbs 25.5g, Fat 10g

CREAMY CUBAN FU FU

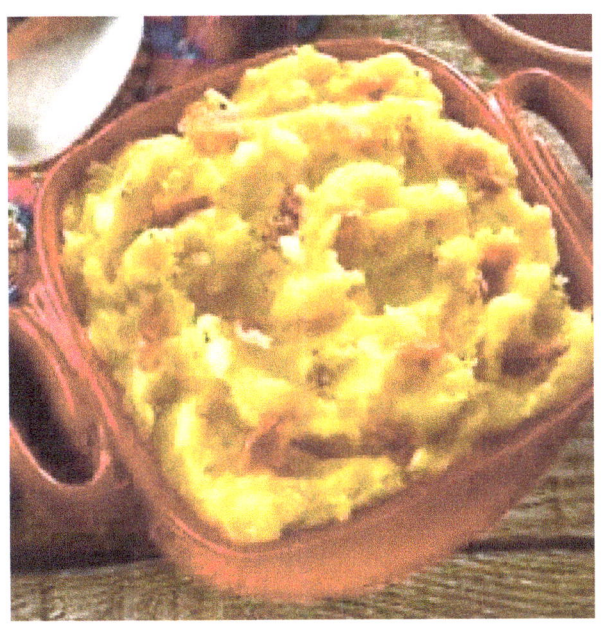

Preparation time: 5 minutes
Cooking time: 15 minutes

Servings: 8

Ingredients:

- 4 slices of Chopped Bacon
- 4 Sliced Sweet Plantains
- 1 Small Chopped Onion
- 1/2 cup of Light Mayonnaise
- 1 clove of Chopped Garlic

Directions:

1. Cover your plantains with water in a 4-quart sauce pot. Bring the pot to a boil over a medium-high heat. Reduce the heat and allow to simmer for approximately 10 minutes until the plantains are tender. Drain the water from your pot and mash your plantains. Set to the side.
2. Cook your bacon in a 10-inch skillet over a medium heat until the bacon is crisp. Drain excess liquid. Reserve a tablespoon of the bacon drippings.
3. Heat your reserved drippings in the same skillet and cook your onion approximately 4 minutes. Make sure to occasionally stir. Once the onion is tender, add your garlic and cook approximately 1 more minute.
4. Combine your plantains, onion mixture, 1/2 of the bacon, and mayonnaise in a serving bowl. Garnish it with your remaining bacon.
5. Serve and Enjoy!

Nutrition Values: calories 266, fat 13.9g, fiber 11.1g, carbs 23.8g, protein 17.5g

ROASTED ASPARAGUS PROSCIUTTO & EGG

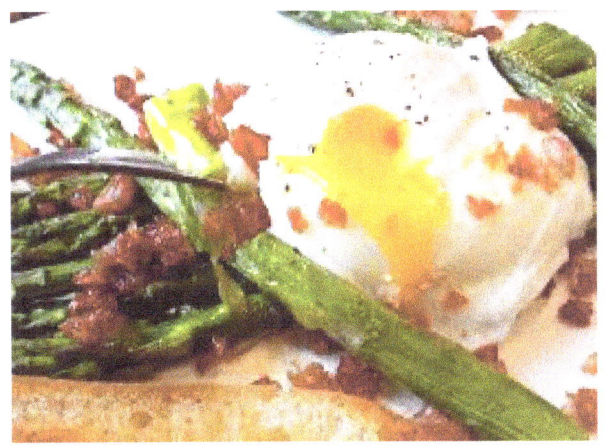

Preparation time: 5 minutes
Cooking time: 20 minutes
Servings: 4

. . .

Ingredients:

- 1 bunch of Trimmed Fresh Asparagus
- 1 tablespoon of Olive Oil
- 1 tablespoon of Extra-Virgin Olive Oil
- 2 ounces of Minced Prosciutto
- 4 Eggs
- 1 teaspoon of Distilled White Vinegar
- 1/2 of a Lemon (Juiced & Zested)
- Pinch of Ground Black Pepper
- Pinch of Salt

Directions:

1. Preheat your oven to 425 degrees.
2. Place your asparagus in a baking dish and then drizzle with your extra-virgin olive oil.
3. Heat olive oil in your skillet over a medium-low heat. Add in your prosciutto. Cook approximately 3 to 4 minutes. Stir it until it is golden colored and rendered. Sprinkle your oil and prosciutto over your asparagus. Season with your pepper and toss it to coat well.
4. Roast it in your oven for approximately 10 minutes. Take out and toss it again.
5. Place back in your oven for an additional 5 minutes until asparagus is firm yet still tender.
6. Fill a big saucepan with approximately 2 to 3 inches of water and boil over a high heat. Reduce the heat to medium-low. Pour in your vinegar and salt.
7. Crack egg into a bowl and then slip your egg gently into the water. Continue this with all of your remaining eggs. Poach your eggs until the whites are firm and the yolks have gotten thick but not hard. Should take approximately 4 to 6 minutes.
8. Remove your eggs using a slotted spoon. Dab on a towel to help remove any excess water. Move to a warm plate.

9. Drizzle lemon juice over asparagus. Place asparagus on plate and top with your poached egg and a pinch of the lemon zest. Season it with your black pepper.
10. Serve and Enjoy!

Nutrition Values: calories 266, fat 13.9g, fiber 11.1g, carbs 23.8g, protein 17.5g

CREAMY LOADED MASHED POTATOES

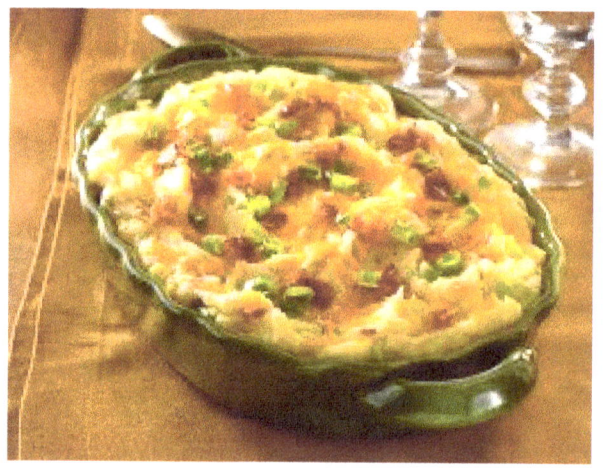

Preparation time: 5 minutes
Cooking time: 45 minutes
Servings: 8

. . .

Ingredients:

- 3 pounds of Cubed and Peeled Potatoes
- 1 cup of Mayonnaise
- 1 cup of Sour Cream
- 6 slices of Bacon or Turkey Bacon
- 1 1/2 cups of Shredded Cheddar Cheese
- 3 Chopped Green Onions

Directions:

1. Cover your potatoes with water in a 4-quart sauce pot. Boil over a high heat. Reduce heat to low and cook approximately 10 minutes until the potatoes are tender. Drain them and mash.
2. Preheat your oven to 375 degrees. Spray baking dish with cooking spray.
3. Stir in mayonnaise, green onions, 4 strips of crumbled bacon, and sour cream. Turn them into your baking dish and cook approximately 30 minutes.
4. Top with remaining 1/2 cup of cheese and your bacon. Bake for 5 more minutes until the cheese has melted.
5. Serve and Enjoy!

Nutrition Values: Calories 202, Protein 2.5g, Carbs 25.5g, Fat 10g

POTATO AND ZUCCHINI OMELET

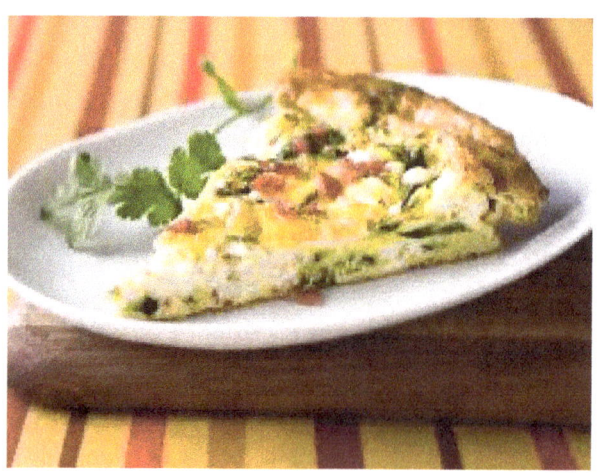

Preparation time: 5 minutes
Cooking time: 10 minutes
Servings: 3

. . .

Ingredients:

- ½ lb. potato (about 1¼ cups diced)
- ½ lb. zucchini (about 1½ cups diced)
- ⅔ cup chopped onion (1 small)
- 1 Tbs. butter
- 2 Tbs. olive oil
- ¼ tsp. dried dill weed
- ¼ tsp. dried basil, crushed
- ½ tsp. crushed dried red pepper
- salt to taste
- fresh-ground black pepper to taste
- 5 to 6 eggs
- butter for frying
- garnish
- sour cream

Directions:

1. Peel or scrub the potato and cut it in ½-inch dice. Wash, trim, and finely dice the zucchini. Drop the diced potato into boiling salted water and cook for 5 minutes, then drain it and set it aside. Cook the diced zucchini in boiling water for 3 to 4 minutes, drain, and set aside.
2. Heat the butter and the olive oil in a medium-sized skillet and sauté the onions in it until they start to color.
3. Add the partially cooked potato and zucchini, the dill weed, basil, crushed red pepper, and salt. Cook this mixture over medium heat, stirring often, until the potatoes are just tender. Grind in some black pepper and add more salt if needed.
4. Make either 2 medium-sized or 3 small omelets according to the directions. When the eggs are almost set, spoon some of the hot vegetables onto one side and fold the other side of the omelet over the filling. Slide the omelets out onto warm plates and serve immediately with sour cream.

Nutrition Values: calories 400, fat 32g, fiber 0g, carbs 2g, protein 24g

SECRET BREAKFAST SUNDAES

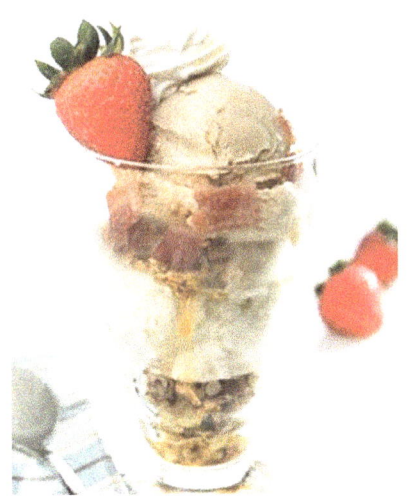

Preparation time: 5 minutes
Cooking time: 10 minutes
Servings: 4

Ingredients:

- 6 slices of Bacon
- 1/2 cup of Heavy Whipping Cream
- 5 tablespoons of Pure Maple Syrup or Pancake Syrup
- 3 tablespoons of Light Brown Sugar
- 3/4 cup of Granola Cereal
- 2 cups of Coffee Ice Cream
- 2 cups of Butter Pecan Ice Cream
- 4 Fresh Strawberries

Directions:

1. Preheat your oven to 400 degrees.
2. Arrange your bacon on a non-stick baking sheet. Sprinkle 1/2 of your brown sugar over the bacon. Bake for approximately 6 minutes. Turn the bacon and sprinkle the remaining brown sugar over it. Bake for an additional 6 minutes until bacon is dark brown. Remove from your oven and allow to cool on a wire rack. Once your bacon has cooled, crumble it up and set it aside.
3. Beat together a tablespoon of maple syrup with a 1/2 cup of cream in a 2-quart metal bowl using an electric mixer. Beat until stiff peaks form and then set aside.
4. Spoon 2 tablespoons of granola into 4 parfait glasses. Evenly scoop the butter pecan ice cream into glasses and sprinkle them with your remaining granola. Add your coffee ice cream to each glass and evenly drizzle the remaining maple syrup on top. Sprinkle with your bacon, and top with strawberries.
5. Serve and Enjoy!

Nutrition Values: Calories 202, Protein 2.5g, Carbs 25.5g, Fat 10g

BANANA NUT OATMEAL

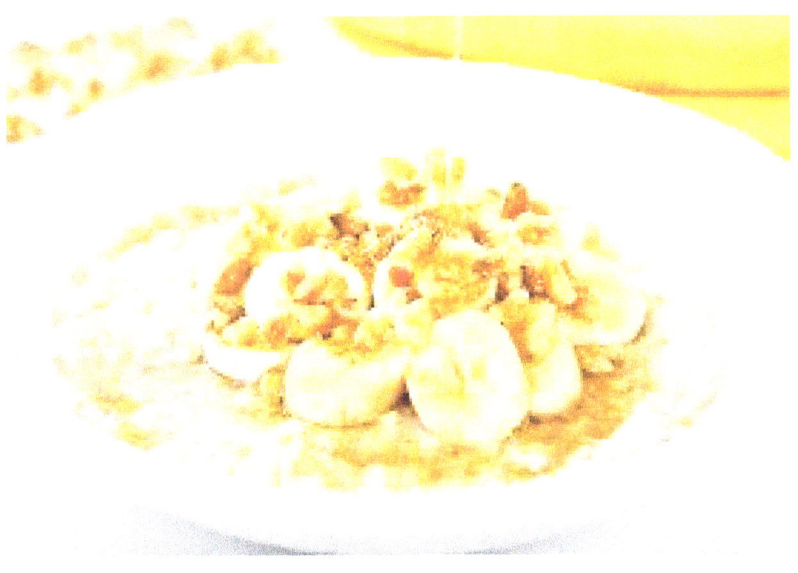

Preparation time: 1 minutes
Cooking time: 2 minutes
Servings: 1

. . .

Ingredients:

- 1 Peeled Banana
- 1/2 cup of Skim Milk
- 1/4 cup of Quick Cooking Oats
- 3 tablespoons of Honey
- 2 tablespoons of Chopped Walnuts
- 1 teaspoon of Flax Seeds

Directions:

1. Combine your milk, oats, honey, walnuts, banana, and flax seeds in a microwave safe bowl. Cook in your microwave for 2 minutes on high. Mash your banana using a fork and stir it into the mixture.
2. Serve and Enjoy!

Nutrition Values: Calories 202, Protein 2.5g, Carbs 25.5g, Fat 10g

GREEK FRITTATA W/ ZUCCHINI, TOMATOES, FETA, AND HERBS

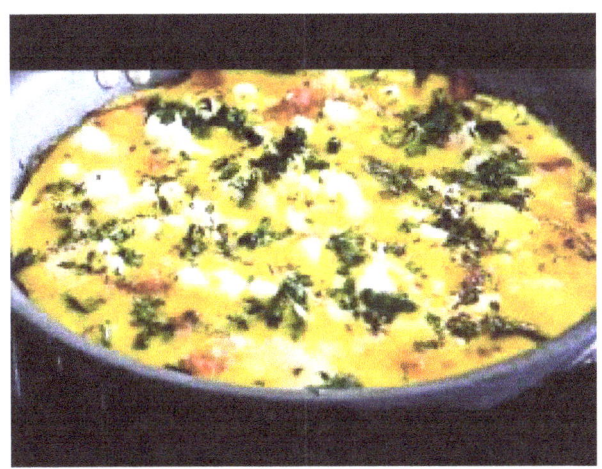

Preparation time: 5 minutes
Cooking time: 10 minutes
Servings: 4

. . .

Ingredients:

- 6 Eggs
- 15 ounces of Diced Tomatoes
- 1 Diced Medium Zucchini
- 1 tablespoon of Olive Oil
- 2 cloves of Minced Garlic
- 1/2 cup of Mozzarella Cheese
- 1 tablespoon of Cream
- 1/4 cup of Crumbled Feta Cheese
- 1/4 teaspoon of Oregano
- 1/2 teaspoon of Dried Basil
- 1 teaspoon of Spike Seasoning
- Cracked Black Pepper

Directions:

1. Pour your tomatoes into your colander and allow them to drain out any liquid into your sink. Cut the ends of your zucchini and dice it into smaller pieces.
2. Preheat your broiler. Spray a frying pan with cooking spray. Heat olive oil in your pan. Add the garlic, zucchini, spike seasoning, and dried herb. Saute them for approximately 3 minutes. Add your tomatoes and cook an additional 3 to 5 minutes. All the liquid from your tomatoes should be evaporated.
3. While your vegetables are cooking, break your eggs in a bowl and beat them well. Pour your eggs into the pan with your vegetable mix and cook an additional 2 to 3 minutes. Eggs should just be beginning to set.
4. Add half of your feta and mozzarella cheese. Stir them in gently. Cook approximately 3 minutes. Sprinkle the rest of your feta and mozzarella cheese over top and allow to cook for 3 more minutes with a lid covering your pan. Cheese should be mostly melted and the eggs should be nearly set.
5. Place under your broiler until the top becomes browned

slightly. Should only take a few minutes. Keep a close eye on it. Rotate the pan if necessary to get an even browning.
6. Sprinkle any additional fresh herbs if you so desire. Cut into pie shaped wedges.
7. Serve and Enjoy!

Nutrition Values: Calories 300, Protein 2.5g, Carbs 25.5g, Fat 10g

GREEK YOGURT PANCAKES

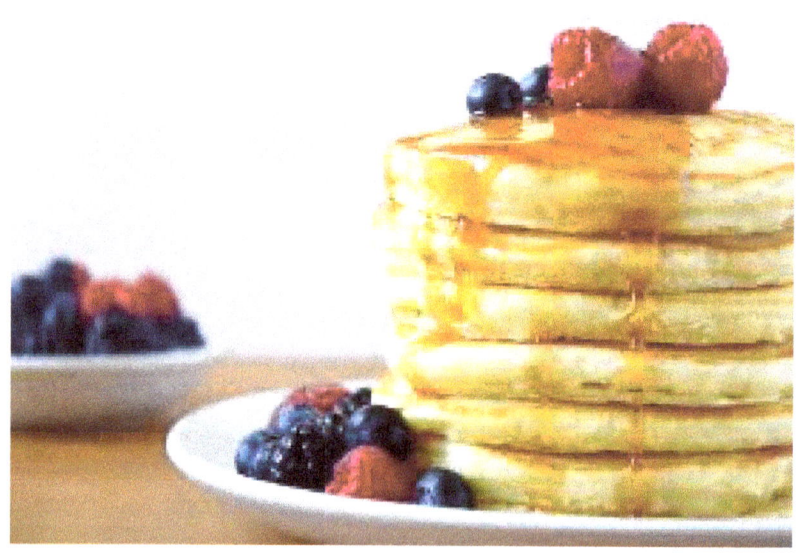

Preparation time: 5 minutes
Cooking time: 25 minutes
Servings: 4

. . .

Ingredients:

- 1 cup of Old-Fashioned Oats
- 2 tablespoons of Flax Seeds
- 1 teaspoon of Baking Soda
- 1/2 cup of All Purpose Flour
- 1/4 teaspoon of Salt
- 2 cups of Vanilla Greek Yogurt
- 2 tablespoons of Honey or Agave
- 2 Large Eggs
- 2 tablespoons of Canola Oil
- Syrup
- Fresh Fruit

Directions:

1. Combine oats, seeds, flour, baking soda, and salt in your blender and pulse for approximately 30 seconds.
2. Add in your eggs, yogurt, agave, and oil. Blend until it is smooth. Let your batter stand approximately 20 minutes in order to thicken.
3. Heat your skillet over a medium heat. Brush your skillet with oil. Ladle your batter 1/4 of a cup at a time into your skillet. Cook your pancakes until the bottoms turn golden brown and bubbles begin forming on top. Should take about 2 minutes. Turn over your pancakes and cook until the bottoms are golden brown. Should take another 2 minutes.
4. Transfer pancakes to your baking sheet. Keep warm in your oven. Repeat process until all your batter is cooked.
5. Add on desired syrup and fruit toppings.
6. Serve and Enjoy!

Nutrition Values: calories 301, fat 5.9g, fiber 11.9g, carbs 26.4g, protein 22.4g

MEDITERRANEAN TOFU SCRAMBLE

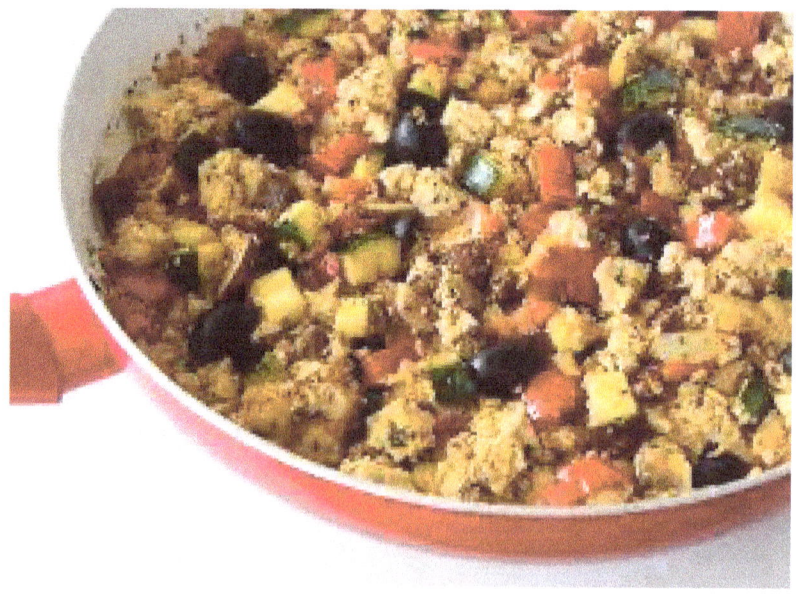

Preparation time: 5 minutes
Cooking time: 10 minutes
Servings: 4

Ingredients:

- 2 tablespoons of Olive Oil
- 1 Diced Purple Onion
- 2 cloves of Minced Garlic
- 1 pound of Extra Firm Tofu
- 1 Diced Medium Red Bell Pepper
- 1 tablespoon of Lemon Juice
- 2 tablespoons of Soy Sauce
- 2 tablespoons of Seasoning
- 1 teaspoon of Ground Turmeric
- 1/4 cup of Finely Chopped Fresh Parsley
- 3 Chopped Scallions
- 1/2 teaspoon of Red Pepper Flakes
- Toast
- Hot Sauce
- Pita Bread
- Hummus

Directions:

1. Coat bottom of your large skillet with olive oil and put it over a medium heat. Once the oil is hot, add your onion and saute until it has softened. Should take about 5 minutes. Add your garlic and cook an additional minute.
2. Crumble the tofu into your skillet and add your soy sauce, bell pepper, seasoning, lemon juice, and red pepper flakes. Keep cooking, flipping with your spatula, until your bell pepper pieces are crisp and tender. Should take about 5 minutes. Remove from the heat and fold in your scallions and parsley.
3. Serve with pita, toast, hot sauce, and hummus. Enjoy!

Nutrition Values: Calories 202, Protein 2.5g, Carbs 25.5g, Fat 10g

Part Two

LUNCH

SMOKED SALMON AND VEGGIES MIX

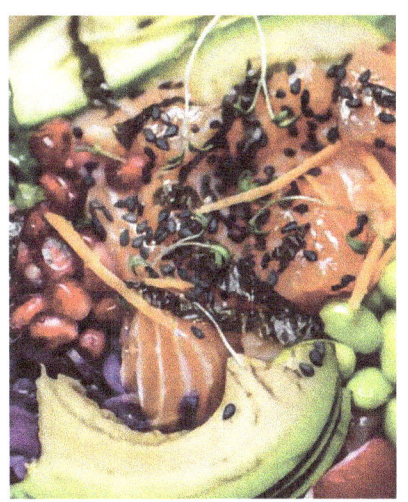

Preparation time: 10 minutes
Cooking time: 20 minutes
Servings: 4

. . .

Ingredients:

- red onions, cut into wedges
- ¾ cup green olives, pitted and halved
- red bell peppers, roughly chopped
- ½ teaspoon smoked paprika
- Salt and black pepper to the taste
- tablespoons olive oil
- salmon fillets, skinless and boneless
- tablespoons chives, chopped

Directions:

1. In a roasting pan, combine the salmon with the onions and the rest of the ingredients, introduce in the oven and bake at 390 degrees F for 20 minutes.
2. Divide the mix between plates and serve.

Nutrition Values: calories 301, fat 5.9g, fiber 11.9g, carbs 26.4g, protein 22.4g

SALMON AND CREAMY ENDIVES

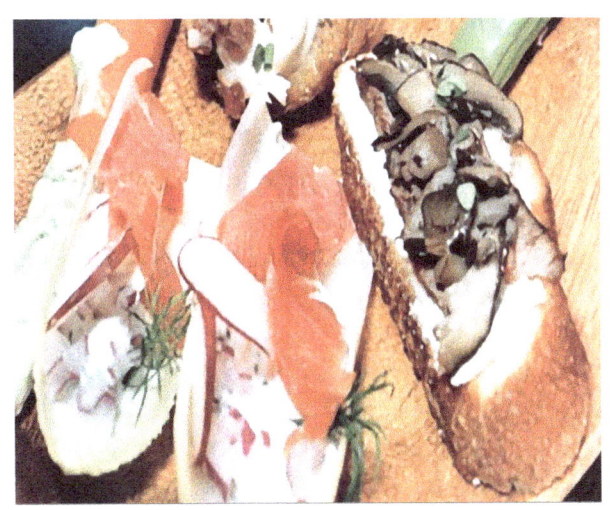

Preparation time: 10 minutes
Cooking time: 15 minutes
Servings: 4

Ingredients:

- salmon fillets, boneless
- endives, shredded
- Juice of 1 lime
- Salt and black pepper to the taste
- ¼ cup chicken stock
- cup Greek yogurt
- ¼ cup green olives pitted and chopped
- ¼ cup fresh chives, chopped
- tablespoons olive oil

Directions:

1. Heat up a pan with half of the oil over medium heat, add the endives and the rest of the ingredients except the chives and the salmon, toss, cook for 6 minutes and divide between plates.
2. Heat up another pan with the rest of the oil, add the salmon, season with salt and pepper, cook for 4 minutes on each side, add next to the creamy endives mix, sprinkle the chives on top and serve.

Nutrition Values: calories 266, fat 13.9g, fiber 11.1g, carbs 23.8g, protein 17.5g

BAKED TROUT AND FENNEL

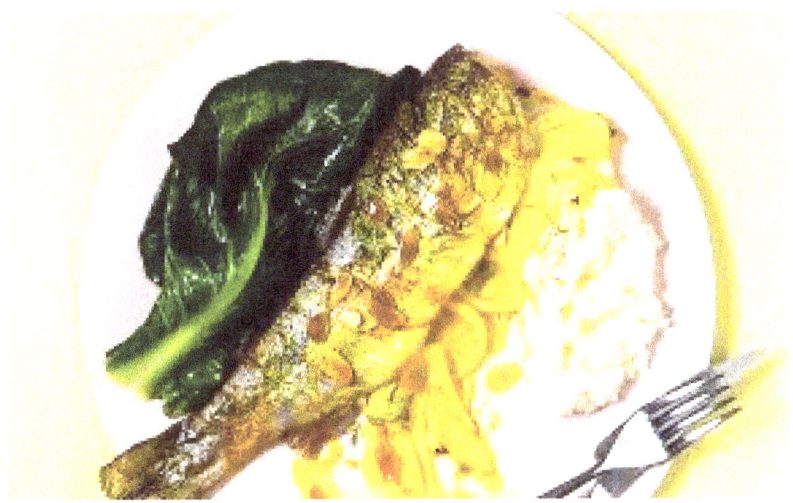

Preparation time: 10 minutes
Cooking time: 22 minutes
Servings: 4

. . .

Ingredients:

- fennel bulb, sliced
- tablespoons olive oil
- yellow onion, sliced
- teaspoons Italian seasoning
- rainbow trout fillets, boneless
- ¼ cup panko breadcrumbs
- ½ cup kalamata olives, pitted and halved
- Juice of 1 lemon

Directions:

1. Spread the fennel the onion and the rest of the ingredients except the trout and the breadcrumbs on a baking sheet lined with parchment paper, toss them and cook at 400 degrees F for 10 minutes.
2. Add the fish dredged in breadcrumbs and seasoned with salt and pepper and cook it at 400 degrees F for 6 minutes on each side.
3. Divide the mix between plates and serve.

Nutrition Values: calories 306, fat 8.9g, fiber 11.1g, carbs 23.8g, protein 14.5g

LAMB STEAK PITA BREADS

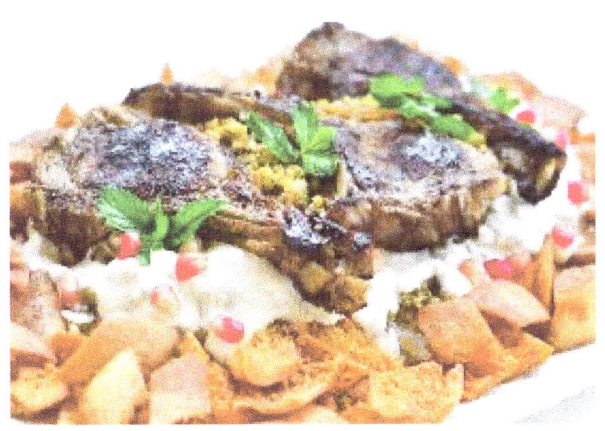

Preparation time: 10 minutes
Cooking time: 10 minutes
Servings: 4

. . .

Ingredients:

- 4 lamb leg steaks
- 1 teaspoon cumin, ground
- 2 teaspoons olive oil
- 1 tablespoon sugar
- 2 carrots, grated
- 3 tablespoons wine vinegar
- 2 spring onions, chopped
- 4 ounces white cabbage, shredded
- 5 sweet peppers
- 4 pita bread
- 3 tablespoons mayonnaise
- Salt and black pepper to taste

Directions:

1. Rub lamb with olive oil, cumin, salt and pepper, place on preheated grill pan over medium high heat, cook for 4 minutes on each side, transfer to a plate and leave aside for now.
2. In a bowl, mix sugar with vinegar and whisk well. Add carrots, cabbage, onion, salt and pepper and toss everything to coat.
3. In a food processor, mix peppers and mayonnaise and blend well.
4. Divide carrots and cabbage mix on each flatbread, add sliced lamb on top and drizzle mayonnaise mix at the end. Roll up flatbreads and serve right away.

Nutrition Values: calories 264, fat 4g, fiber 2g, carbs 5g, protein 9g

BAKED LAMB WITH EGGPLANT AND GREEK YOGURT

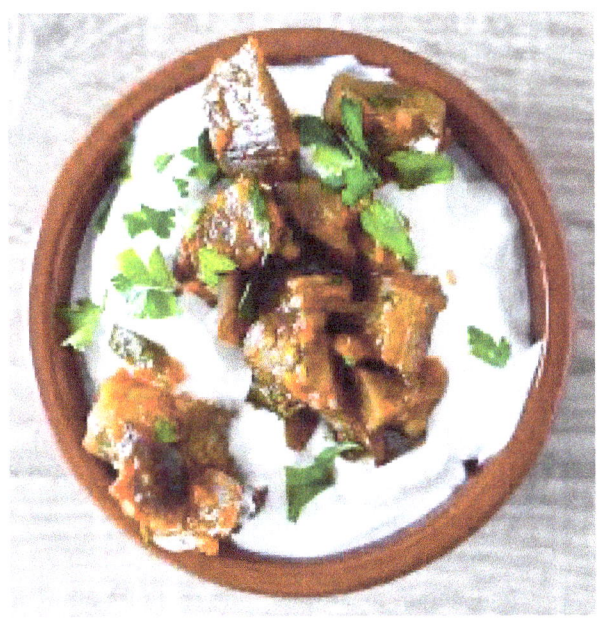

PREPARATION TIME: 15 MINUTES

Cooking time: 1 hour
Servings: 6

Ingredients:

- 4 eggplants, cut into halves lengthwise
- 4 ounces olive oil
- 2 yellow onions, chopped
- 4 ounces lamb meat, ground
- 2 green bell peppers, chopped
- 1 pound tomatoes, chopped
- 4 tomato slices
- 2 tablespoons tomato paste
- ½ cup parsley, chopped
- 4 garlic cloves, minced
- ½ cup hot water
- Greek yogurt for serving
- Salt and pepper to taste

Directions:

1. Heat a pan with the olive oil over medium high heat, add eggplant halves, cook for 5 minutes, flipping once and transfer to a plate.
2. Heat the same pan over medium high heat, add onion, stir and cook for 3 minutes.
3. Add bell peppers and cook for 2 more minutes. Add lamb, tomato paste, salt, pepper and chopped tomatoes and stir again. Add parsley and cook for 5 more minutes.
4. Place eggplant halves on a baking tray, open them up, divide garlic in each, spoon meat filling and top with a tomato slice.
5. Pour water over them, cover tray with foil and bake in the oven at 350 degrees F for 40 minutes.

6. Take out of the oven, transfer to plates and serve with yogurt on top.

Nutrition Values: calories 253, fat 3g, fiber 2g, carbs 5g, protein 10g

BEEF STEAKS WITH SPICY SAUCE

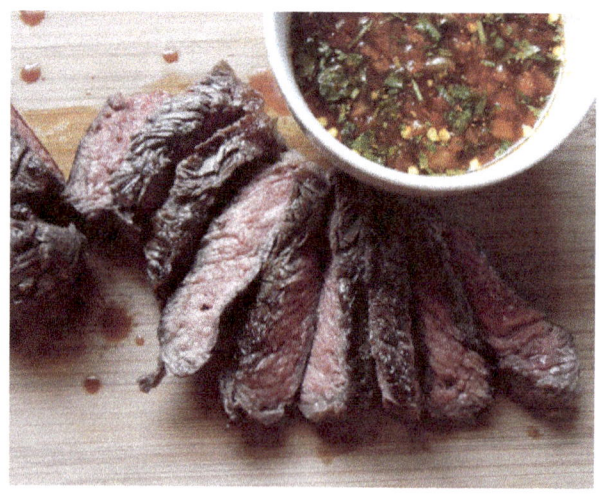

Preparation time: 10 minutes
Cooking time: 15 minutes
Servings: 4

Ingredients:

- 2 teaspoons chili powder
- 2 and ½ tablespoons olive oil
- Salt and black pepper to taste
- 1 ½ teaspoons onion powder
- 1 ½ teaspoons garlic powder
- 1 tablespoon smoked paprika
- 1 red bell pepper, cut in halves
- 2 tomatoes, cut in halved
- 1 small red onion, cut into 6 wedges
- 4 beef steaks
- 2 teaspoons sherry vinegar
- 1 tablespoon oregano, chopped
- Hot sauce to taste
- A pinch of cumin, ground
- 1/3 cup black olives, pitted and sliced

Directions:

1. In a bowl, mix chili powder with paprika, salt, pepper, garlic and onion powder.
2. In another bowl, mix bell pepper with onion, tomatoes, 1 tablespoon spice mixture and ½ tablespoon oil then toss to coat.
3. Mix steaks with remaining spice mix and toss to coat. Heat your kitchen grill pan over medium high heat, add pepper and onion, cook for 4 minutes on each side and transfer to a plate.
4. Add tomatoes, grill for 2 minutes and also transfer to the plate with the rest of the veggies.
5. Place steaks on the grill, cook for 4 minutes on each side and transfer to a platter. In a blender, mix grilled veggies with cumin, remaining oil, vinegar, oregano, salt, pepper and hot sauce and blend until you obtain a sauce.
6. Serve steaks with this sauce on top and with chopped olives.

Nutrition Values: calories 450, fat 23g, fiber 2g, carbs 8g, protein 43g

DELICIOUS SAUSAGE KEBABS

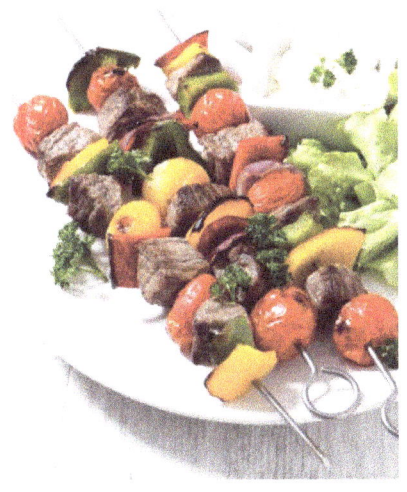

Preparation time: 1 hour
Cooking time: 13 minutes
Servings: 6

. . .

Ingredients:

- 1 yellow onion, chopped
- 1 pound ground pork
- 3 tablespoons parsley, chopped
- 1 tablespoon lemon juice
- 1 garlic clove, minced
- 1 teaspoon oregano, dried
- 1 teaspoon mint, dried
- Salt and black pepper to taste
- Vegetable oil

For the sauce:

- 2 tablespoons olive oil
- ¼ cup tahini sauce
- ¼ cup water
- 1 tablespoon lemon juice
- 1 garlic clove, minced
- Salt and cayenne pepper to taste

Directions:

1. In a bowl, mix ground pork with onion, parsley, 1 garlic clove, 1 tablespoon lemon juice, mint, oregano, salt and pepper to taste, stir well and divide into 6 portions.
2. Shape your kebabs by squeezing each portion on a skewer, cover and keep them in the fridge for 1 hour.
3. Heat your kitchen grill pan over medium high heat, place kebabs on it, brush them with vegetable oil, cook them for 13 minutes, turning from time to time and transfer to plates.
4. In a food processor, mix tahini with olive oil, 1 tablespoon lemon juice, 1 garlic clove, water, salt and cayenne pepper and blend well.
5. Serve your kebabs with this sauce all over.

Nutrition Values: calories 250, fat 23g, fiber 1g, carbs 4g, protein 14g

TURKEY CUTLETS

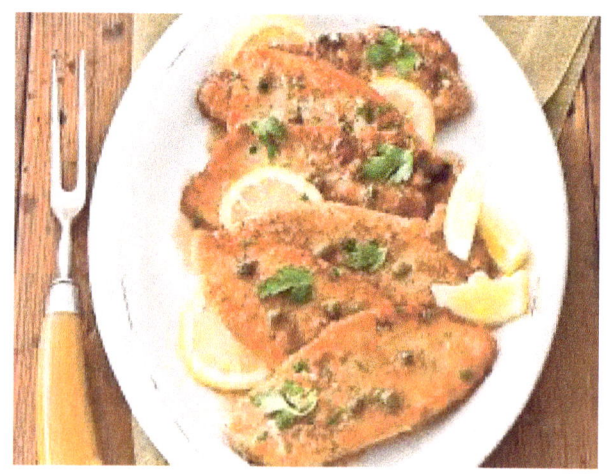

Preparation time: 10 minutes
Cooking time: 25 minutes
Servings: 4

. . .

Ingredients:

- 1 ½ cups couscous
- ½ cup vegetable oil
- 1 cup breadcrumbs
- 2 cups chicken stock
- 1 tablespoons sesame seeds
- Salt and black pepper to taste
- A pinch of paprika
- A pinch of cayenne pepper
- 2 eggs
- 4 turkey breast cutlets
- ¼ cup parsley, chopped
- 4 ounces feta cheese, crumbled
- ¼ cup red onion, chopped
- ½ cup white flour
- 4 lemon wedges

Directions:

1. Heat a pan with 2 tablespoon oil over medium high heat, add couscous, stir and cook for 7 minutes.
2. Add stock, bring to a boil, reduce heat to medium-low, simmer for 10 minutes, take off heat and keep warm.
3. In a bowl, mix breadcrumbs with sesame seeds, cayenne, paprika, salt and pepper. Whisk eggs well in another bowl and put the flour in a third one.
4. Dredge turkey cutlets in flour, eggs and breadcrumbs and arrange on the plate.
5. Heat a pan with remaining oil over medium high heat, add cutlets, cook for 3 minutes flipping once and transfer them to paper towels in order to drain excess grease.
6. Mix couscous with parsley onion, salt, pepper and feta cheese and stir.
7. Divide turkey cutlets on plates, add couscous on the side and serve with lemon wedges.

Nutrition Values: calories 760, fat 20g, fiber 4g, carbs 34, protein 40g

SLOW COOKED CHICKEN

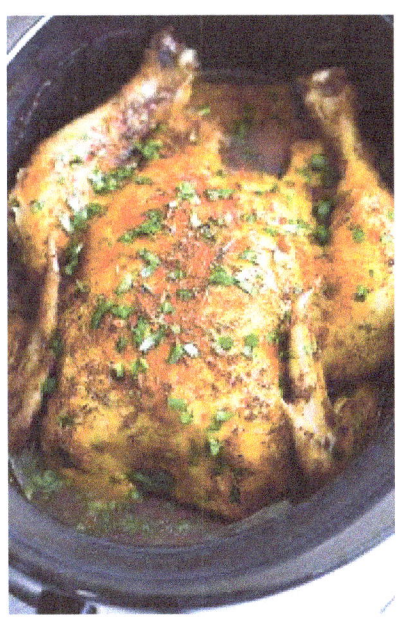

Preparation time: 10 minutes
Cooking time: 6 hours and 15 minutes

Servings: 4

Ingredients:

- 1 pound carrots, roughly chopped
- Zest from 1 lemon
- 30 apricots, dried
- ¼ cup white flour
- ¼ teaspoon cinnamon, ground
- A pinch of ginger, ground
- ¼ teaspoon coriander, ground
- A pinch of cardamom, ground
- Salt and black pepper to taste
- A pinch of cayenne pepper
- 8 chicken thighs, bone-in and skinless
- 2 tablespoons vegetable oil
- 2 and ¼ cups yellow onion, chopped
- 2 tablespoons tomato paste
- 1 tablespoon butter
- 1 and ½ tablespoons garlic, minced
- ¼ cup lemon juice
- 1 cup apricot juice
- ½ cup chicken stock
- ¼ cup cilantro, chopped
- ¼ cup pine nuts, toasted

Directions:

1. Add lemon peel, apricots and carrots to a slow cooker. In a bowl, mix flour with salt, pepper, cayenne pepper, cinnamon, coriander, ginger and cardamom.
2. Add chicken pieces and toss to coat well. Heat a pan with the oil and butter over medium-high heat, add chicken pieces and brown for 11 minutes.

3. Transfer to the slow cooker. Add garlic and onion to the heated pan, stir and cook for 3 minutes.
4. Add tomato paste, stock, nectar and lemon juice, stir, bring to a boil, simmer for 2 minutes and pour into your slow cooker.
5. Cook everything for 6 hours on High, transfer to plates, garnish with nuts and cilantro on top.

Nutrition Values: calories 340, fat 3g, fiber 4g, carbs 12g, protein 20g

MEDITERRANEAN MEATLOAF

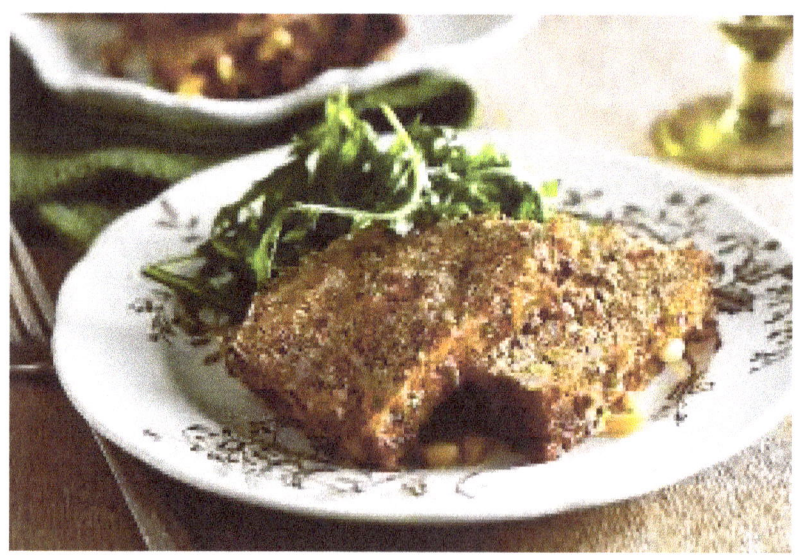

Preparation time: 10 minutes
Cooking time: 1 hour and 20 minutes
Servings: 8

. . .

Ingredients:

- 1 yellow onion, chopped
- 2 tablespoons olive oil
- 2 garlic cloves, minced
- ¾ cup red wine
- 4 ounces white bread, chopped
- 2 pounds lamb, ground
- 1 cup milk
- ¼ cup feta cheese, crumbled
- 2 eggs
- 1/3 cup kalamata olives, pitted and chopped
- 4 tablespoons oregano, chopped
- Salt and black pepper to taste
- 2 tablespoons honey
- 1 tablespoon Worcestershire sauce
- 2 teaspoons lemon zest, grated

Directions:

1. Heat a pan with 2 tablespoons oil over medium heat, add garlic and onion, stir and cook for 8 minutes.
2. Add wine, stir, simmer for 5 minutes and transfer everything to a bowl.
3. Put bread pieces in a bowl, add milk, leave aside for 10 minutes, squeeze bread a bit, chop and add it to onions mix.
4. Add lamb, eggs, cheese, olives, lemon, zest, oregano, Worcestershire sauce, salt and pepper to onions mix and stir well.
5. Transfer meatloaf mix to a baking dish, spread honey all over, place in the oven at 375 degrees F and bake for 50 minutes.
6. Take meatloaf out of the oven, leave aside for 5 minutes, slice and arrange on a platter.

Nutrition Values: calories 350, fat 23g, fiber 1g, carbs 17g, protein 24g

CHILI CALAMARI AND VEGGIE MIX

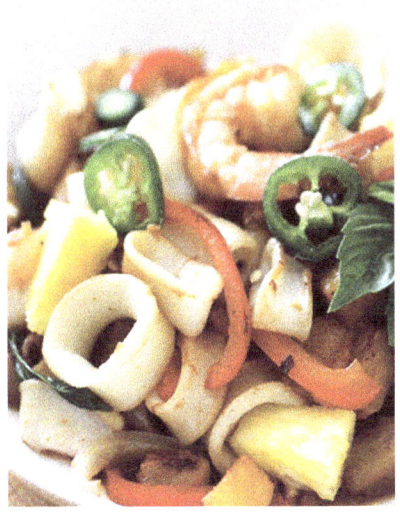

Preparation time: 10 minutes
Cooking time: 40 minutes
Servings: 4

. . .

Ingredients:

- pound calamari rings
- red chili peppers, chopped
- tablespoons olive oil
- garlic cloves, minced
- 14 ounces canned tomatoes, chopped
- 2 tablespoons tomato paste
- tablespoon thyme, chopped
- Salt and black pepper to the taste
- tablespoons capers, drained
- 12 black olives, pitted and halved

Directions:

1. Heat up a pan with the oil over medium-high heat, add the garlic and the chili peppers and sauté for 2 minutes.
2. Add the rest of the ingredients except the olives and capers, stir, bring to a simmer and cook for 22 minutes.
3. Add the olives and capers, cook everything for 15 minutes more, divide everything into bowls and serve.

Nutrition Values: calories 274, fat 11.6g, fiber 2.8g, carbs 13.5g, protein 15.4g

GREEK TROUT SPREAD

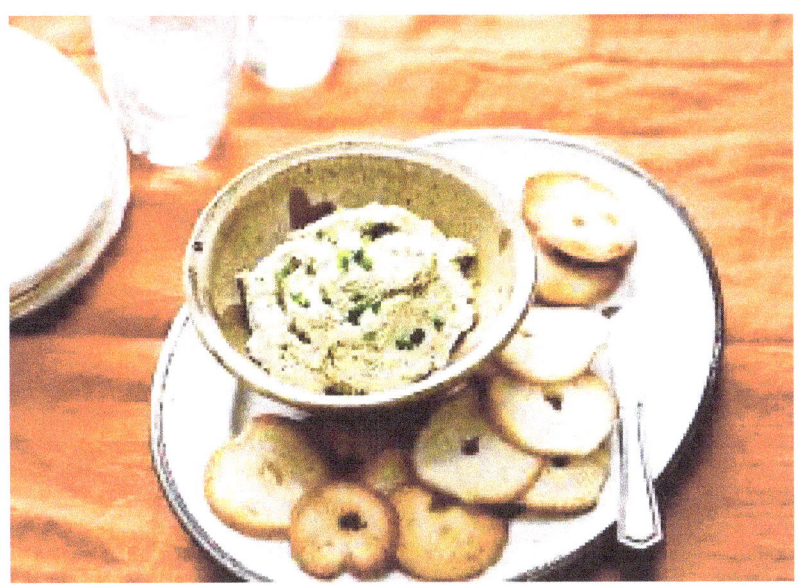

Preparation time: 5 minutes
Cooking time: 0 minutes
Servings: 8

Ingredients:

- 4 ounces smoked trout, skinless, boneless and flaked
- tablespoon lemon juice
- 1 cup Greek yogurt
- tablespoon dill, chopped
- Salt and black pepper to the taste
- A drizzle of olive oil

Directions:

1. In a bowl, combine the trout with the lemon juice and the rest of the ingredients and whisk really well.
2. Divide the spread into bowls and serve.

Nutrition Values: calories 258, fat 4,5g, fiber 2g, carbs 5.5g, protein 7.6g

CAYENNE COD AND TOMATOES

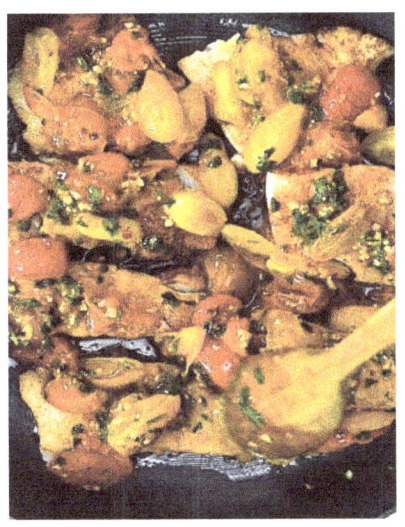

Preparation time: 10 minutes
Cooking time: 25 minutes
Servings: 4

. . .

Ingredients:

- teaspoon lime juice
- Salt and black pepper to the taste
- teaspoon sweet paprika
- teaspoon cayenne pepper
- tablespoons olive oil yellow onion, chopped
- garlic cloves, minced
- cod fillets, boneless
- A pinch of cloves, ground
- ½ cup chicken stock
- ½ pound cherry tomatoes, cubed

Directions:

1. Heat up a pan with the oil over medium-high heat add the cod, salt, pepper and the cayenne, cook for 4 minutes on each side and divide between plates.
2. Heat up the same pan over medium-high heat, add the onion and garlic and sauté for 5 minutes.
3. Add the rest of the ingredients, stir, bring to a simmer and cook for 10 minutes more.
4. Divide the mix next to the fish and serve.

Nutrition Values: calories 232, fat 16.5g, fiber 11.1g, carbs 24.8g, protein 16.5g

SHRIMP AND DILL MIX

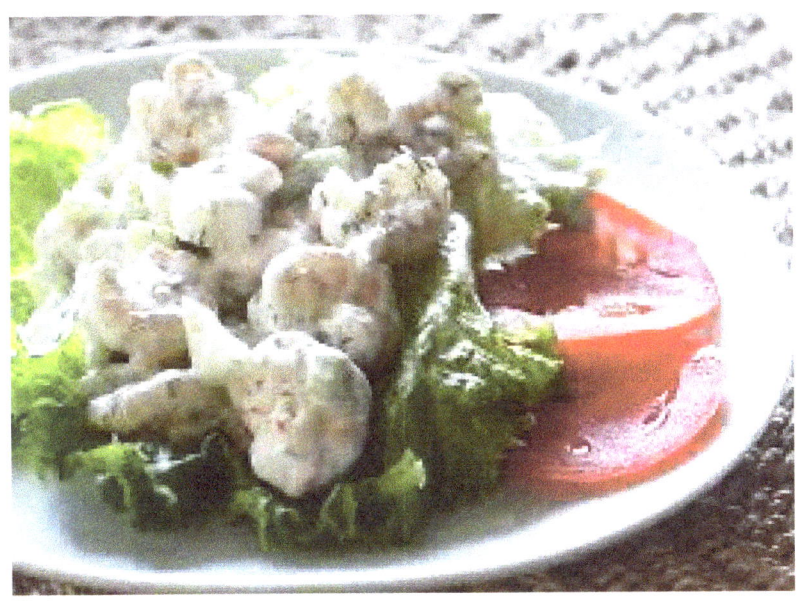

Preparation time: 10 minutes
Cooking time: 10 minutes
Servings: 4

Ingredients:

- pound shrimp, cooked, peeled and deveined
- ½ cup raisins cup spring onion, chopped
- tablespoons olive oil
- tablespoons capers, chopped
- tablespoons dill, chopped
- Salt and black pepper to the taste

Directions:

1. Heat up a pan with the oil over medium-high heat, add the onions and raisins and sauté for 2-3 minutes.
2. Add the shrimp and the rest of the ingredients, toss, cook for 6 minutes more, divide between plates and serve with a side salad.

Nutrition Values: calories 218, fat 12.8g, fiber 6.2g, carbs 22.2g, protein 4.8g

SALMON & ASPARAGUS

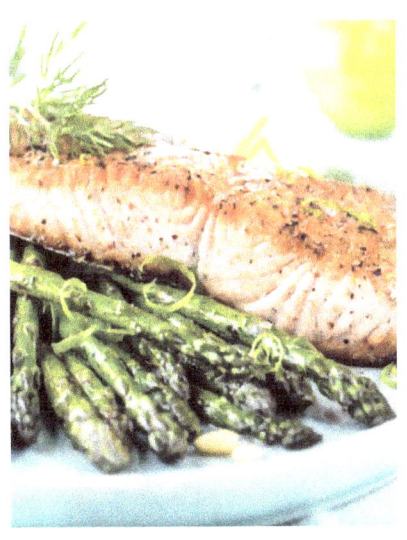

Preparation time: 3 minutes
Cooking time: 10 minutes
Servings: 3

. . .

Ingredients:

- 1 lb. Salmon Fillets
- 10 Ounces Asparagus, Fresh
- 1 Sprig Rosemary, Fresh
- ½ Cup Cherry Tomatoes, Halved
- 1 Tablespoon Olive Oil mixed with 1 Tablespoon Lemon Juice

Directions:

1. Add in a cup of water and then add in your steamer basket.
2. Place your salmon fillets onto the rack and then add in your rosemary. Top with asparagus.
3. Cover the pot, and then cook on high pressure for three minutes.
4. Use a quick release, and serve drizzled with dressing and with your tomatoes on the side.

Nutrition Values: calories 267, protein 31.7g, fat 14.3 g, carbs 5.2 g, cholesterol 67 mg

HIGH-QUALITY BELIZEAN CHICKEN STEW

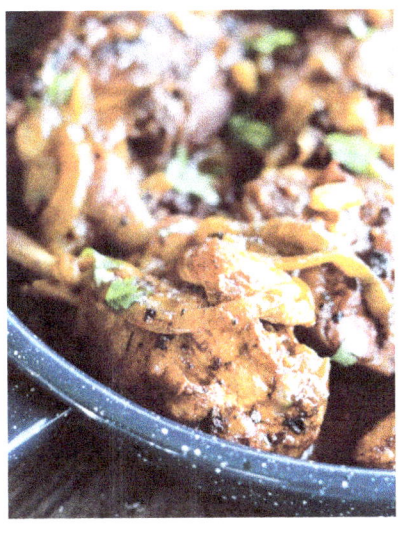

Preparation time: 5 minutes
Cooking time: 25 minutes
Servings: 4

. . .

Ingredients

- 1 whole chicken
- 1 tablespoon coconut oil
- 2 tablespoons achiote seasoning
- 2 tablespoons white vinegar
- 3 tablespoons Worcestershire sauce
- 1 cup yellow onion, sliced
- 3 garlic cloves, sliced
- 1 teaspoon ground cumin
- 1 teaspoon dried oregano
- ½ teaspoon black pepper
- 2 cups chicken stock

Directions

1. Take a large sized bowl and add achiote paste, vinegar, Worcestershire sauce, oregano, cumin and pepper. Mix well and add chicken pieces and rub the marinade all over them
2. Allow the chicken to sit overnight. Set your pot to Saute mode and add coconut oil
3. Once the oil is hot, add the chicken pieces to the pot and brown them in batches (each batch for 2 minutes). Remove the seared chicken and transfer them to a plate
4. Add onions, garlic to the pot and Saute for 2-3 minutes. Add chicken pieces back to the pot
5. Pour chicken broth to the bowl with marinade and stir well. Add the mixture to the pot
6. Seal up the lid and cook for about 20 minutes at high pressure
7. Once done, release the pressure naturally. Season with a bit of salt and serve!

Nutrition Values: calories 218, fat 12.8g, fiber 6.2g, carbs 22.2g, protein 4.8g

THE GREAT POBLANO CHICKEN CURRY

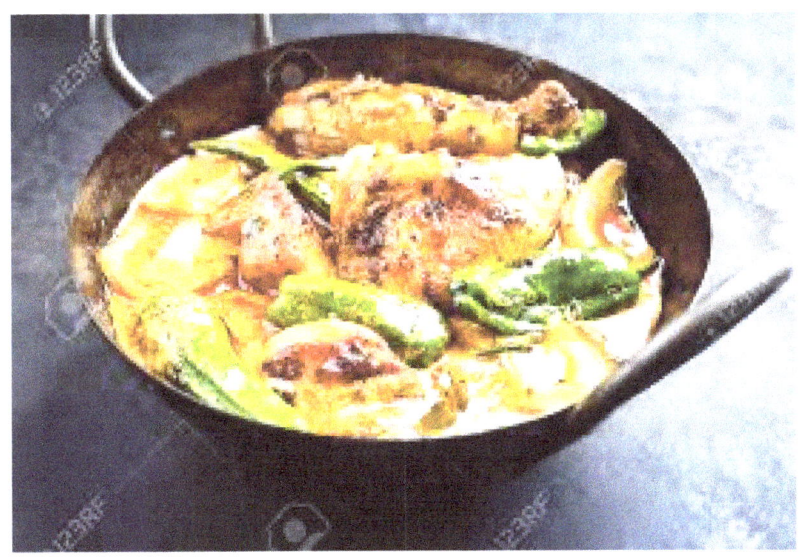

Preparation time: 5 minutes
Cooking time: 30 minutes
Servings: 4

. . .

Ingredients

- 1 cup onion, diced
- 3 poblano peppers, chopped
- 1 and ½ pounds large chicken breast chunks
- ¼ cup cilantro, chopped
- 1 teaspoon ground coriander
- 1 teaspoon ground cumin
- 1-2 teaspoons salt
- 2 and ½ cups of water
- 2 ounces cream cheese

Directions

1. Add everything to your Ninja Foodi except cheese and lock up the lid
2. Cook on HIGH pressure for 15 minutes. Release the pressure naturally over 10 minutes
3. Remove the chicken with tongs and place it on the side
4. Use an immersion blender to blend the soup and veggies. Set your pot to Saute mode
5. Once the broth is hot add cream cheese (Cut in chunks). Whisk well
6. Shred the chicken and transfer it back to the pot. Serve and enjoy!

Nutrition Values: calories 218, fat 12.8g, fiber 6.2g, carbs 22.2g, protein 4.8g

THE ORIGINAL MEXICAN CHICKEN CACCIATORE

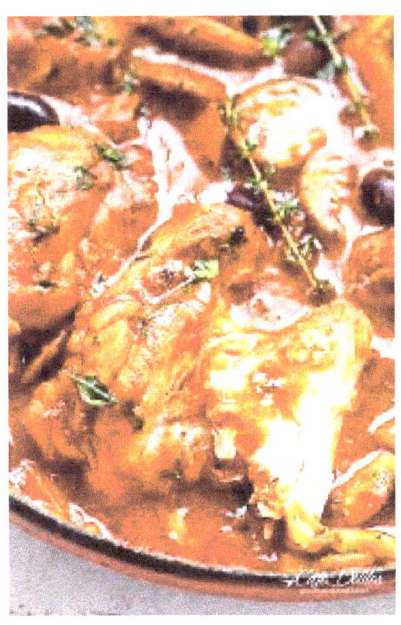

PREPARATION TIME: 5 MINUTES
COOKING TIME: 50 MINUTES

Servings: 4

Ingredients

- Extra virgin olive oil'
- 3 shallots, chopped
- 4 garlic cloves, crushed
- 1 green bell pepper, sliced
- ½ cup organic chicken broth
- 10 ounces mushrooms, sliced
- 5-6 skinless chicken breasts
- 2 cans (14.5 ounces) organic crushed tomatoes
- 2 tablespoons organic tomato paste
- 1 can (14.5 ounces) black olives, pitted
- Fresh parsley
- Salt and pepper to taste

Directions

1. Add oil to your pot and set the Ninja Foodi to Saute mode
2. Add shallots, bell pepper and cook for 2 minutes
3. Add broth and bring to a boil for 23 minutes. Add garlic and mushrooms
4. Gently place the chicken on the top of the whole mixture
5. Cover the chicken with tomato paste and crushed tomatoes
6. Lock up the lid and cook on HIGH pressure for 8 minutes
7. Release the pressure naturally over 10 minutes and stir in parsley, olive oil, pepper, salt, and red pepper flakes. Serve!

Nutrition Values: calories 340, fat 3g, fiber 4g, carbs 12g, protein 20g

MAGNIFICENT CHICKEN CURRY SOUP

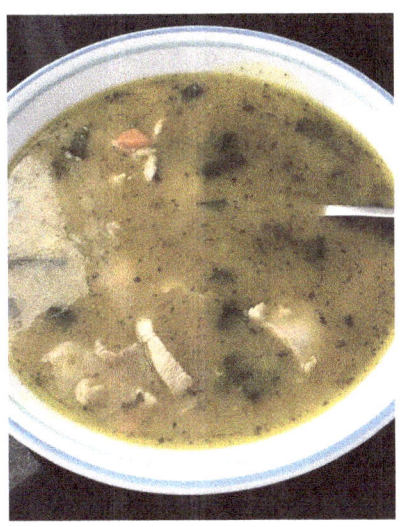

Preparation time: 5 minutes
Cooking time: 20 minutes
Servings: 4

Ingredients

- 1 and ½ cups unsweetened coconut milk
- 1 pound chicken thigh, skinless
- 3-4 garlic cloves, crushed
- ½ an onion, finely diced
- 2-inch knob ginger, minced
- 1 cup mushrooms, sliced
- 4 ounces baby spinach
- ½ teaspoon of cayenne pepper
- ½ teaspoon turmeric
- 1 teaspoon salt
- 1 teaspoon Garam Masala
- ¼ cup cilantro, chopped

Directions

1. Add the listed ingredients to Ninja Foodi
2. Lock lid and cook on HIGH pressure for 10 minutes. Naturally, release pressure over 10 minutes
3. Remove meat and shred it, return the shredded meat to the pot
4. Set your pot to Saute mode and stir for a minute
5. Serve and enjoy!. Enjoy!

Nutrition Values: calories 258, fat 4.5g, fiber 2g, carbs 5.5g, protein 7.6g

AWESOME LIGURIAN CHICKEN

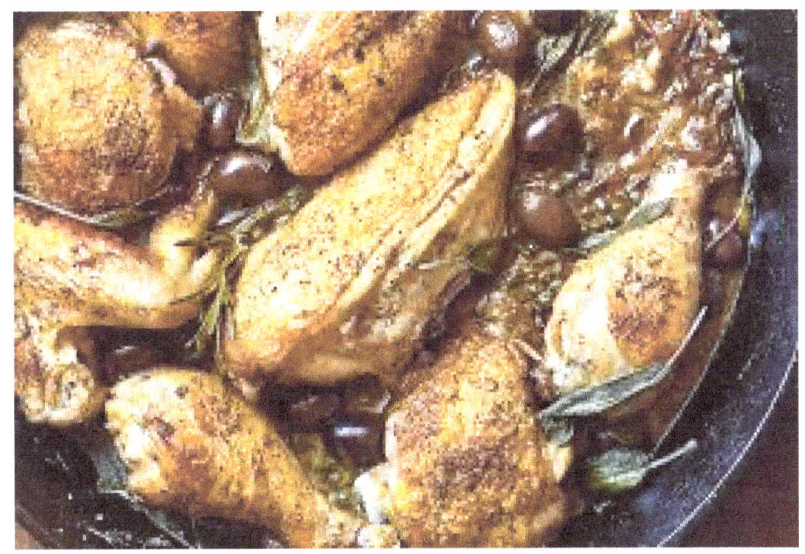

Preparation time: 5 minutes
Cooking time: 4 hours 10 minutes
Servings: 4

. . .

Ingredients

- 2 garlic cloves, chopped
- 3 sprigs fresh rosemary
- 2 sprigs fresh sage
- ½ bunch parsley
- 3 lemon, juiced
- 4 tablespoons extra virgin olive oil
- 1 teaspoon salt
- ¼ teaspoon pepper
- 1 and ½ cup of water
- 1 whole chicken, cut into parts
- 3 and ½ ounces black gourmet salt-cured olives
- 1 fresh lemon

Directions

1. Take a bowl and add chopped up garlic, parsley, sage, and rosemary
2. Pour lemon juice, olive oil to a bowl and season with salt and pepper
3. Remove the chicken skin and from the chicken pieces and carefully transfer them to a dish
4. Pour the marinade on top of the chicken pieces and allow them to chill for 2-4 hours
5. Set your Ninja Foodi to Saute mode and add olive oil, allow it to heat up. Add chicken and browned on all sides
6. Measure out the marinade and add to the pot (it should cover the chicken, add a bit of water if needed). Lock up the lid and cook on HIGH pressure for 10 minutes
7. Release the pressure naturally. The chicken out and transfer to a platter
8. Cover with a foil and allow them to coolSet your pot in Saute mode and reduce the liquid to ¼
9. Add the chicken pieces again to the pot and allow them to warm

10. Sprinkle a bit of olive, lemon slices, and rosemary. Enjoy!

Nutrition Values: calories 274, fat 11.6g, fiber 2.8g, carbs 13.5g, protein 15.4g

GARLIC AND LEMON CHICKEN DISH

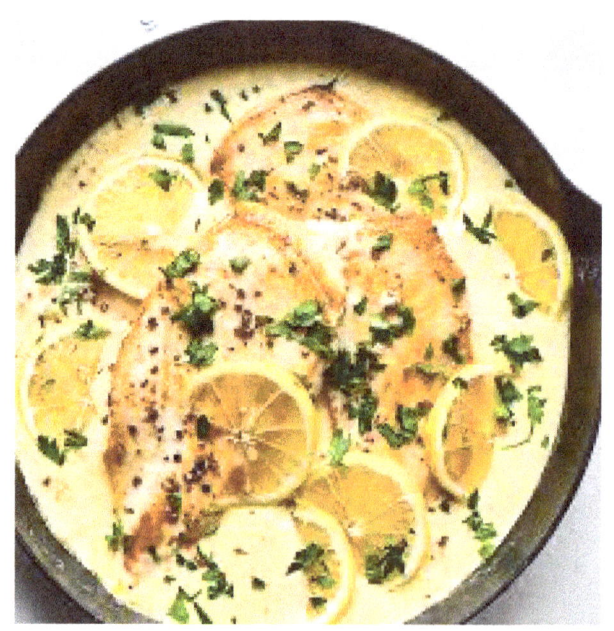

Preparation time: 5 minutes
Cooking time: 30 minutes

Servings: 4

Ingredients

- 2-3 pounds chicken breast
- 1 teaspoon salt
- 1 onion, diced
- 1 tablespoon ghee
- 5 garlic cloves, minced
- ½ cup organic chicken broth
- 1 teaspoon dried parsley
- 1 large lemon, juiced
- 3-4 teaspoon arrowroot flour

Directions

1. Set your pot to Saute mode. Add diced up onion and cooking fat
2. Allow the onions to cook for 5 -10 minutes
3. Add the rest of the ingredients except arrowroot flour
4. Lock up the lid and set the pot to poultry mode. Cook until the timer runs out
5. Allow the pressure to release naturally
6. Once done, remove ¼ cup of the sauce from the pot and add arrowroot to make a slurry
7. Add the slurry to the pot to make the gravy thick. Keep stirring well. Serve!

Nutrition Values: calories 340, fat 3g, fiber 4g, carbs 12g, protein 20g

Part Three

DINNER

GARLIC SHRIMP WITH OLIVE OIL

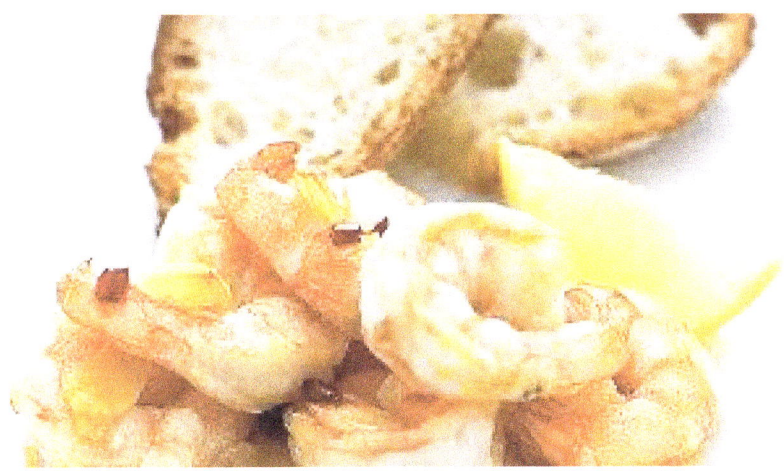

Preparation time: 4 minutes
Cooking time: 10 minutes
Servings: 5

. . .

Ingredients:

- 1 cup extra-virgin oil
- 4 garlic cloves, minced
- 6 whole dried red chilies
- ¼ cup minced flat-leaf parsley
- 2 pound shelled and deveined medium shrimp
- Pinch of salt
- Crusty bread, for serving (optional)

Directions:

1. Heat olive oil in a very large deep skillet until shimmering.
2. Then, add the garlic, chilies, and parsley and cook over moderately high heat for 10 seconds, stirring.
3. Add on the shrimp and cook over high heat, stirring once, until they are pink and curled 3 to 4 minutes.
4. Season with salt and pepper to taste. Transfer to small bowls.
5. Serve with crusty bread. Enjoy!

Each serving contains: Calories 175, Total Fat 2.2g, Protein 32g, Carbohydrate 8.3g, Cholesterol 80mg

STEAMED MUSSELS IN TOMATO GARLIC

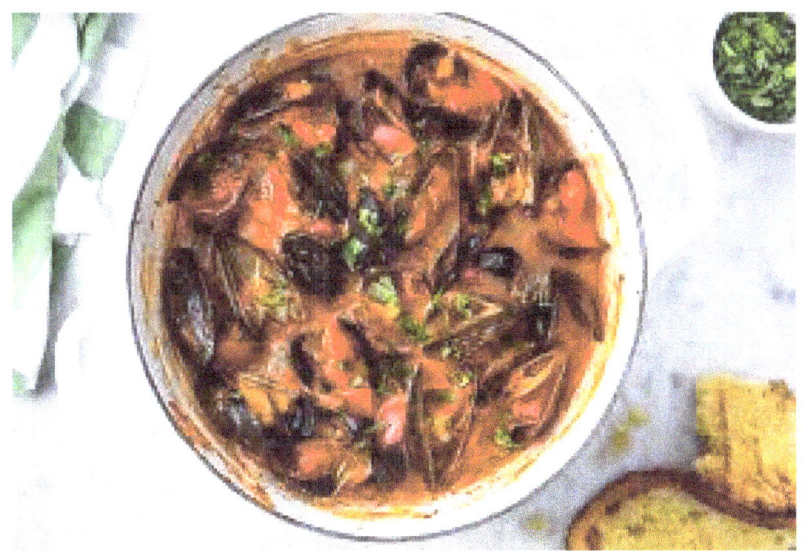

Preparation time: 5 minutes
Cooking time: 23 minutes
Servings: 4

. . .

Ingredients:

- ¼ cup olive oil
- 1 medium-size onion, finely chopped
- 6 cloves garlic, minced
- 3 tablespoons fresh scallions, chopped
- 2 cups canned tomatoes, chopped
- ¼ teaspoon dried thyme
- ¼ teaspoon dried red-pepper flakes
- 4 pounds' mussels, cleaned
- 1/8 teaspoon freshly ground black pepper
- Pinch of salt to taste
- Crusty bread (optional)

Directions:

1. Prepare a large pot, then heat the oil over moderately low heat.
2. Then add the onion and garlic and cook, stirring occasionally, until the onion is translucent, about 5 minutes.
3. Stir in the scallions, tomatoes, thyme, and red pepper flakes.
4. Reduce the heat and simmer, partially covered, for 15 minutes, stirring occasionally.
5. Add the mussels to the pot. Cover; bring to a boil.
6. Cook, and stir the pot occasionally, just until the mussels open, about 3 minutes. Remove the open mussels.
7. Continue to boil, uncovering the pot as necessary to remove the mussels as soon as their shells open. Discard any that do not open longer.
8. Stir the black pepper into the broth. Add salt to taste.
9. Ladle the broth over the mussels. Serve in a bowl with crusty bread to sop up the sauce. Enjoy!

Each serving contains: Calories 272, Total Fat 5.2g, Protein 35g, Carbohydrate 12.7g, Cholesterol 25mg

MEDITERRANEAN-STYLE MUSSELS

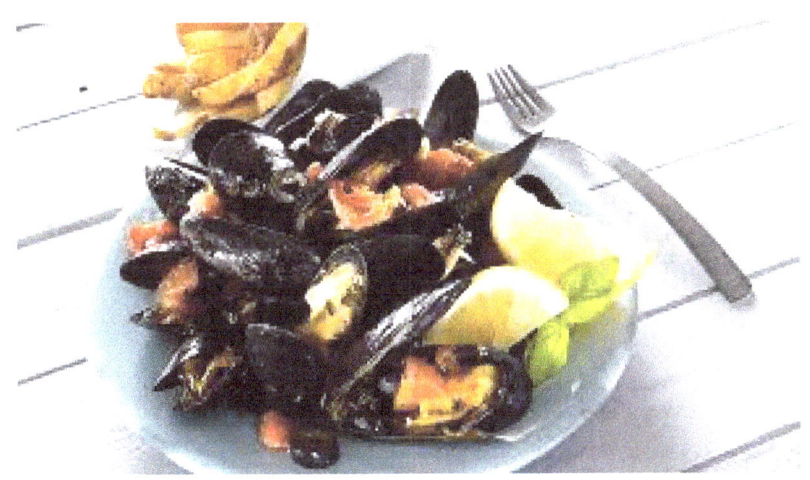

Preparation time: 5 minutes
Cooking time: 21 minutes
Servings: 2

Ingredients:

- 1 medium-size onion, chopped
- 5 cloves garlic, minced
- 1 tablespoon extra-virgin olive oil
- 4 ripe tomatoes, plum
- 1 small size bell pepper
- 1 tablespoon capers, drained
- 1 teaspoon dried oregano
- 500g mussels, cleaned

Directions:

1. Heat oil in a large, wide saucepan over medium heat.
2. Add onion and garlic. Stirring often, cook for 3 min.
3. Meanwhile, coarsely chop tomatoes and pepper. Add to the onion along with capers. Sprinkle with seasonings.
4. Stir often until tomatoes start to break down, 5 to 7 min.
5. Meanwhile, scrub mussels and pull off beards. Discard any that are open. Stir into a thickened tomato mixture.
6. Cover and cook until most mussels open, about 6 min. Stir halfway through cooking.
7. Discard any mussels that are not open after 6 min. Taste and add salt if needed.
8. Serve in wide soup bowls with crusty bread. Enjoy!

Each serving contains: Calories 212, Total Fat 8.3g, Protein 18.2g, Carbohydrate 11.7g, Cholesterol 35mg

LEEKS AND CALAMARI MIX

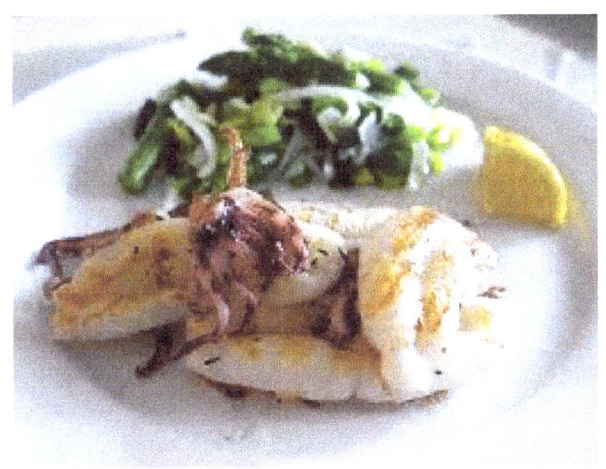

Preparation time: 5 minutes
Cooking time: 15 minutes
Servings: 4

. . .

Ingredients:

- 2 tablespoons avocado oil
- 2 leeks, chopped
- 1 red onion, chopped
- Salt and black to the taste
- 1 pound calamari rings
- 1 tablespoon parsley, chopped
- 1 tablespoon chives, chopped
- 2 tablespoons tomato paste

Directions:

1. Heat a pan with the avocado oil over medium heat, add the leeks and the onion, stir and sauté for 5 minutes.
2. Add the rest of the ingredients, toss, simmer over medium heat for 10 minutes, divide into bowls and serve.

Each serving contains: Calories 238, Total Fat 9g, Protein 8.4g, Carbohydrate 14.4g, Cholesterol 95mg

SEAFOOD PAELLA

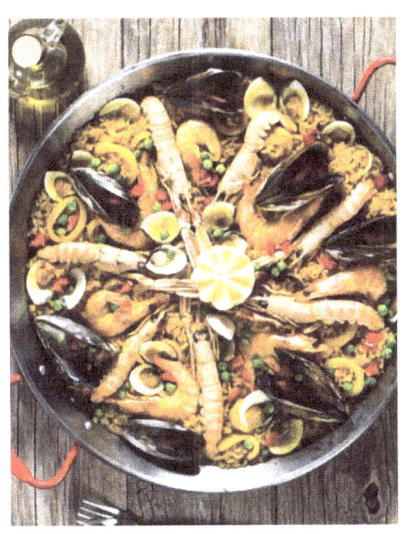

Preparation time: 5 minutes
Cooking time: 35 minutes
Servings: 4

Ingredients:

- 1 tablespoon extra-virgin olive oil
- 4 cloves garlic, minced
- 1 medium-size onion, finely chopped
- 1 red bell pepper, finely chopped
- 300g short or medium grain rice
- ½ teaspoon turmeric
- 1 teaspoon paprika
- 1 14-ounces canned tomatoes, chopped
- 3 cups chicken stock
- 2 pinch of saffron threads
- 12 large shrimp, peeled and deveined
- 12 little neck mussel, thawed
- Handful fresh parsley, roughly chopped
- Lemon wedges

Directions:

1. In a deep pan over medium-high heat, add olive oil, garlic, onion, and red bell pepper and cook for 3 minutes or until vegetables softened.
2. Then, add rice, turmeric, and paprika and stir well. Then add tomatoes, chicken stock and saffron, stir and bring to a boil.
3. Lower heat to simmer and cover and cook for another 20 minutes. Spread shrimp, mussels, and green peas on top.
4. Cover and cook for another 10-15 minutes, until mussels have opened and shrimps are pink.
5. Turn off the heat and sprinkle with parsley on top. Serve with lemon wedges on top. Enjoy!

Each serving contains: Calories 233, Total Fat 5.2g, Protein 13g, Carbohydrate 33g, Cholesterol 18mg

BAKED SALMON IN GARLIC PEPPER

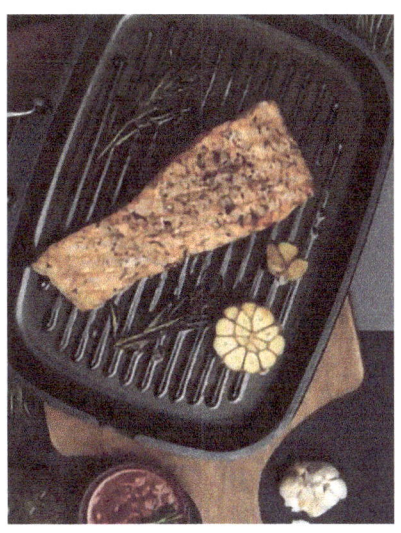

Preparation time: 10 minutes
Cooking time: 25 minutes
Servings: 3

Ingredients:

- 4 (6-ounce) salmon fillets
- 4 tablespoons unsalted butter
- 1 tablespoon garlic, minced
- 3 tablespoons capers, drained
- Fresh herbs like parsley, chives or dill
- Salt and Pepper
- Lemon quartered

Directions:

1. Heat the oven to 325 degrees Fahrenheit. Season both sides of the salmon with salt and pepper.
2. Melt the butter in a wide oven-safe skillet over medium heat.
3. When the butter is bubbling, stir in the garlic and capers. Cook, stirring, until warm, about 1 minute.
4. Take the skillet off of the heat. Add the salmon fillets, skin-side down, to the skillet.
5. Tilt the pan so that butter pools on one side, and then spoon garlic caper butter over each fillet.
6. Cover the skillet with a sheet of aluminum foil or cover with parchment paper by loosely tucking it around the salmon.
7. Bake the salmon, covered, for 15 minutes. Uncover, and then spoon more of the butter over the salmon.
8. Continue to roast, uncovered, until your desired doneness, 5 to 10 minutes more, depending on how thick the salmon is. Tip: We cook salmon until an instant-read thermometer reads 125 degrees Fahrenheit when inserted into the thickest part.
9. Alternatively, you can finish cooking the salmon under the broiler for some extra color on top. Watch closely so the fish does not overcook.
10. Squeeze fresh lemon juice over the baked salmon, sprinkle with lots of fresh herbs.

11. Serve with another spoonful of the garlic caper butter on top. Enjoy!

Each serving contains: Calories 294, Total Fat 11.3g, Protein 28.2g, Carbohydrate 1.7g, Cholesterol 85mg

SAUTEED OCTOPUS

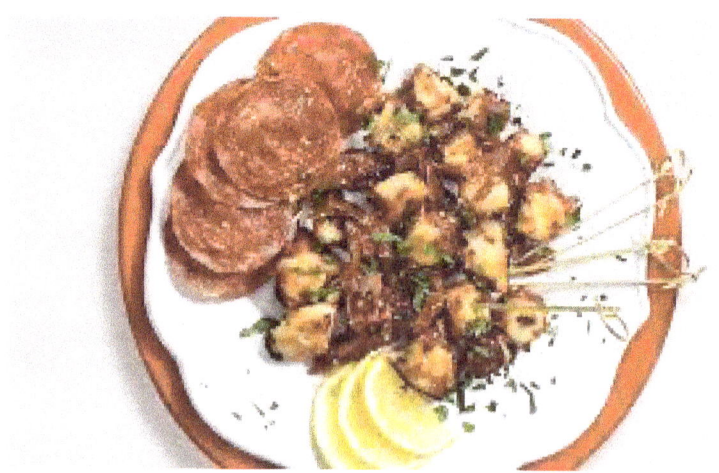

Preparation time: 5 minutes
Cooking time: 1 hour 10 minutes
Servings: 4

. . .

Ingredients:

- 2 pounds' whole octopus, cleaned and cooked ahead (see the Directions below)
- 2 tablespoons extra-virgin olive oil
- 2 medium-size green chili
- 2 plum tomatoes, sliced
- ¼ pitted olives
- 2 tablespoons fresh oregano leaves, chopped
- 2 teaspoons cider vinegar

Directions:

How to cook the whole octopus:

- All frozen octopus is pre-cleaned, and if buying fresh, you can ask the fishmonger to clean it for you.
- In a large stockpot, bring water to a boil and then reduce to a simmer. Add whole octopus, and simmer for 1 hour.
- Remove the octopus from boiling water, and let cool at room temperature for 15 minutes.
- To Sauté: Cut the tentacles from the head, and discard the head. Chop the tentacles into small pieces.
- Heat a large sauté pan with olive oil over medium heat, add the octopus, green chili, tomatoes, olives, oregano, and vinegar.
- Sauté for 10 minutes. Serve immediately.

Each serving contains: Calories 274, Total Fat 8.3g, Protein 35.2g, Carbohydrate 9.8g, Cholesterol 75mg

GRILLED OCTOPUS

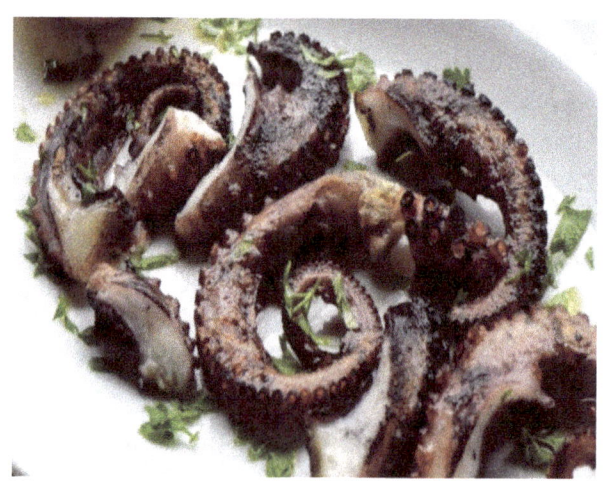

Preparation time: 40 minutes
Cooking time: 1 hour 15 minutes
Servings: 4

Ingredients:

- 1 pound of fresh octopus (medium or large), cleaned and cook ahead
- 1/3 cup freshly squeezed lemon juice
- ¼ cup lemon zest
- 2 garlic heads, minced
- 2 tablespoon parsley, minced
- ½ teaspoon dried oregano
- 2/3 cup Olive oil
- Salt and Pepper, to taste

Directions:

1. Place octopus in a pot and cover with enough water. Bring to boil for 40 minutes.
2. Remove the octopus from hot water, rinse and place in a bowl.
3. Drizzle with olive oil and add chopped garlic. Let it cool and rest at room temperature for 30 minutes to 1 hour.
4. Preheat a gas grill to medium-high heat. Slice octopus's tentacles.
5. Grill for 3-4 minutes per side until charred. Remove from heat and place in a bowl.
6. Drizzle with olive oil and add lemon juice. Season with salt and pepper.
7. Sprinkle some oregano and parsley on top. Add some garlic (optional).
8. Serve and Enjoy!

Each serving contains: Calories 243, Total Fat 6.3g, Protein 38.2g, Carbohydrate 4g, Cholesterol 0mg

SCALLOP SALAD

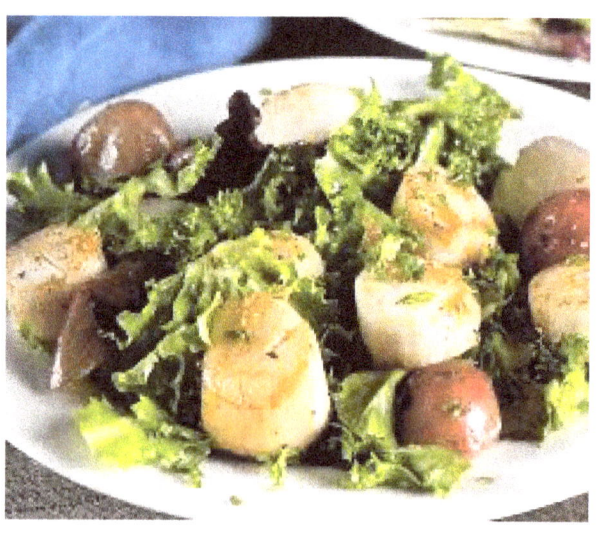

PREPARATION TIME: 15 MINUTES
COOKING TIME: 35 MINUTES
SERVINGS: 6

. . .

Ingredients:

- 12 ounces dry sea scallops
- 4 tablespoons olive oil + 2 teaspoons
- 4 teaspoons soy sauce
- 1 ½ cup quinoa, rinsed
- 2 teaspoons garlic, minced
- A pinch of salt
- 3 cups water
- 1 cup snow peas, sliced
- 1 teaspoon sesame oil
- 1/3 cup rice vinegar
- 1 cup scallions, sliced
- 1/3 cup red bell pepper, chopped
- ¼ cup cilantro, chopped

Directions:

1. In a bowl, mix scallops with 2 teaspoons soy sauce, toss and leave aside for now.
2. Heat a pan with 1 tablespoon olive oil over medium heat, add quinoa, stir and cook for 8 minutes. Add garlic, stir and cook for 1 more minute.
3. Add water and a pinch of salt, bring to a boil, stir, cover and cook for 15 minutes. Add snow peas, cover and leave for 5 more minutes.
4. Meanwhile, in a bowl, mix 3 tablespoons olive oil with 2 teaspoons soy sauce, vinegar and sesame oil and whisk well.
5. Add quinoa and snow peas to mixture and stir again. Add scallions, bell pepper and stir again.
6. Pat dry the scallions and discard marinade. Heat another pan with 2 teaspoons olive oil over medium high heat, add scallions and cook for 1 minute on each side.
7. Add scallops to quinoa salad, stir gently and serve with chopped cilantro on top.

Nutrition Values: Calories 201, Total Fat 5g, Fiber 2g, Carbs 5g, Protein 8g

DELICIOUS CHICKEN SOUP

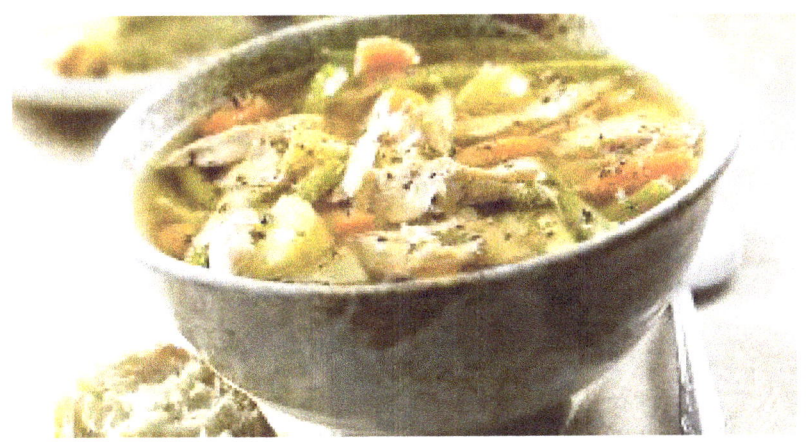

Preparation time: 10 minutes
Cooking time: 1 hour
Servings: 8

. . .

Ingredients:

- 2 cups eggplant, diced
- Salt and black pepper to taste
- ¼ cup olive oil + 1 tablespoon cup yellow
- onion, chopped
- tablespoons garlic, minced
- red bell pepper, chopped
- hot paprika 2 + teaspoons
- ¼ cup parsley, chopped
- teaspoon turmeric
- and ½ tablespoons oregano, chopped
- cups chicken stock pound chicken breast, skinless, boneless and cut into small pieces c
- up half and half and ½ tablespoons cornstarch
- egg yolks
- ¼ cup lemon juice
- Lemon wedges for serving

Directions:

1. In a bowl, mix eggplant pieces with ¼ cup oil, salt and pepper to taste and toss to coat.
2. Arrange eggplant on a lined baking sheet, place in the oven at 400 degrees F and bake for 10 minutes.
3. Flip, cook for 10 minutes more and set aside to cool. Heat a saucepan with 1 tablespoon oil over medium heat, add garlic and onion, cover and cook for 10 minutes.
4. Add bell pepper, stir and cook uncovered for 3 minutes. Add hot paprika, ginger and turmeric and stir well. Add the stock, chicken, eggplant pieces, oregano and parsley.
5. Stir, bring to a boil and simmer for 12 minutes. In a bowl, mix cornstarch with half and half and egg yolks - stir well.
6. Add 1 cup soup, stir again and pour gradually into soup. Stir,

add salt and pepper to taste and lemon juice. Ladle into soup bowls and serve with lemon wedges on the side.

Nutrition Values: Calories 242, Fat 3g, Fiber 2g, Carbs 5g, Protein 3g

CLASSIC MEDITERRANEAN CHICKEN SOUP

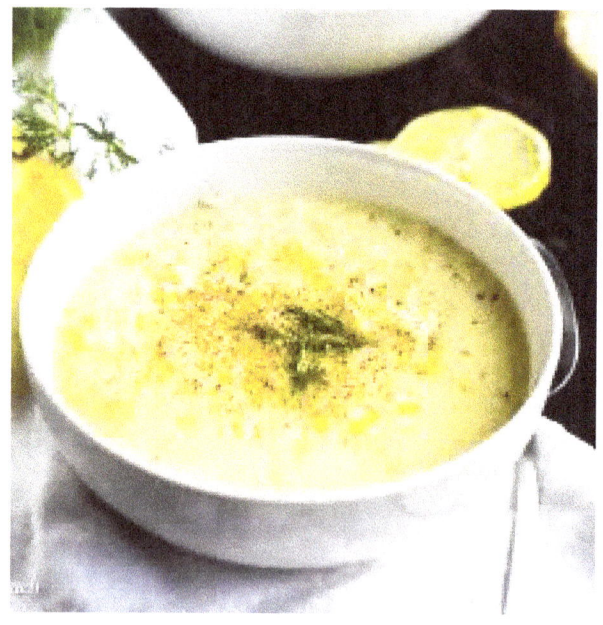

PREPARATION TIME: 15 MINUTES

Cooking time: 1 hour and 20 minutes
Servings: 4

Ingredients:

- big chicken
- tablespoons salt
- cups water leek, cut in quarters
- bay leaves carrot, cut into quarters
- tablespoons olive oil
- 2/3 cup rice
- cups yellow onion, chopped
- eggs ½ cup lemon juice
- teaspoon
- black pepper

Directions:

1. Put chicken in a large saucepan, add water and 2 tablespoons salt, bring to a boil over medium high heat, reduce heat and skim foam.
2. Add carrot, bay leaves and leek and simmer for 1 hour. Heat a pan with the oil over medium high heat, add onion, stir and cook for 6 minutes, take off heat and leave aside for now.
3. Transfer chicken to a cutting board and leave aside to cool down.   Strain soup back into the saucepan.
4. Add sautéed onion and rice, bring again to a boil over high heat, reduce temperature to low and simmer for 20 minutes.
5. Discard chicken bones and skin, dice into big chunks and return to boiling soup.   Meanwhile, in a bowl, mix lemon juice with eggs and black pepper and stir well.
6. Add 2 cups boiling soup and whisk again well.

7. Pour this into the soup and stir well.
8. Add remaining salt, stir, take off heat, transfer to soup bowls and serve right away.

Nutrition Values: Calories 242, Fat 3g, Fiber 2g, Carbs 3g, Protein 3g

EASY CHICKEN STEW

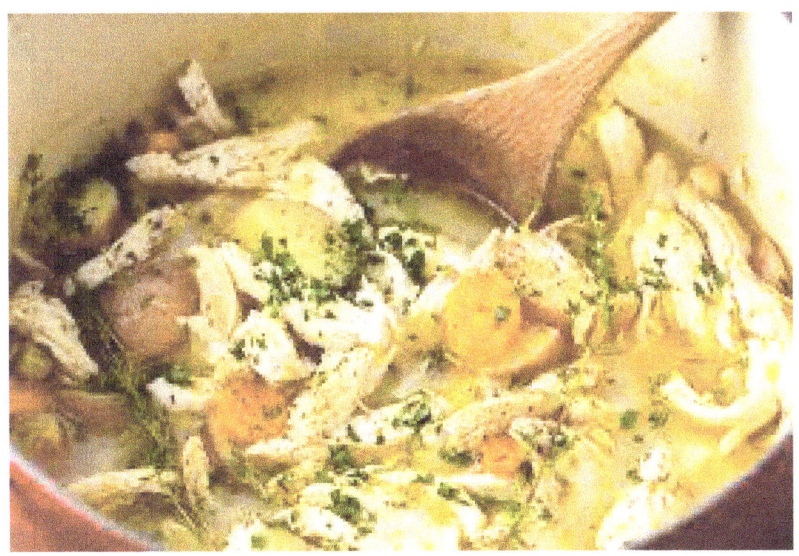

Preparation time: 20 minutes
Cooking time: 40 minutes
Servings: 4

. . .

Ingredients:

- 3 ½ pounds chicken, cut into 10 medium pieces
- 2 yellow onions, chopped
- 2 tablespoons olive oil garlic clove, minced
- ¼ pint chicken stock, warm tablespoon white flour
- teaspoons mixed dried herbs (parsley and basil)
- 14 ounces canned tomatoes, chopped
- Salt and black pepper to taste

Directions:

1. Heat a saucepan with the oil over medium high heat, add chicken meat, stir and brown it for 5 minutes, take off heat, transfer to a plate and set aside.
2. Return saucepan to heat, add garlic and onion, stir and cook for 3 minutes.
3. Add flour and stir well. Add herbs, tomatoes and stock, stir, bring to a boil and season with salt and pepper to taste.
4. Add chicken pieces, stir, reduce heat to medium and simmer the stew for 45 minutes. Transfer to plates and serve right away.

Nutrition Values: Calories 200, Fat 4g, Fiber 3g, Carbs 7g, Protein 12g

CHICKEN AND CABBAGE MIX

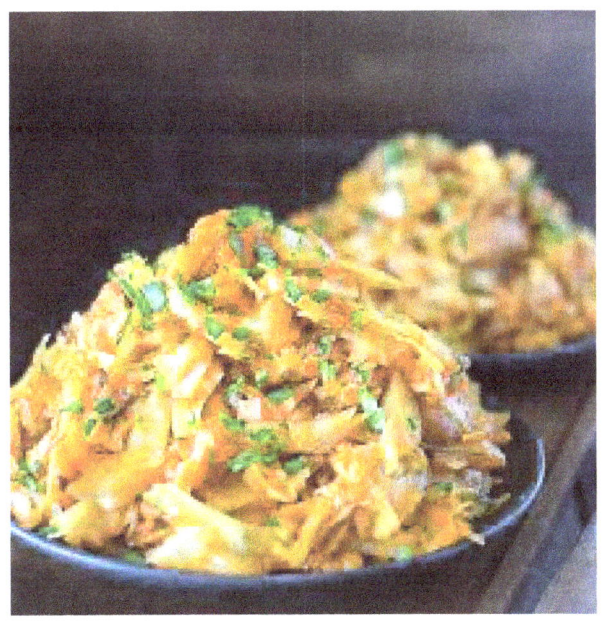

Preparation time: 10 minutes
Cooking time: 6 minutes

Servings: 4

Ingredients:

- 3 medium chicken breasts, skinless, boneless and cut into thin strips
- 4 ounces green cabbage, shredded
- 5 tablespoon extra virgin olive oil
- Salt and black pepper to taste
- 2 tablespoons sherry vinegar tablespoon chives, chopped
- ¼ cup feta cheese, crumbled
- ¼ cup barbeque sauce
- bacon slices, cooked and crumbled

Directions:

1. In a bowl, mix 4 tablespoon oil with vinegar, salt and pepper to taste and stir well.
2. Add the shredded cabbage, toss to coat and leave aside for now.
3. Season chicken with salt and pepper, heat a pan with remaining oil over medium high heat, add chicken, cook for 6 minutes, take off heat, transfer to a bowl and mix well with barbeque sauce.
4. Arrange salad on serving plates, add chicken strips, sprinkle cheese, chives and crumbled bacon and serve right away.

Nutrition Values: Calories 200, Fat 15g, Fiber 3g, Carbs 10g, Protein 33g

MEDITERRANEAN CHICKEN AND RICE SOUP

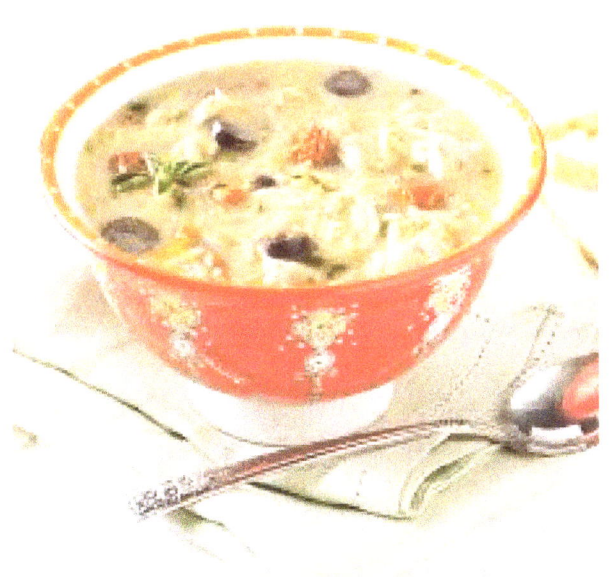

Preparation time: 10 minutes
Cooking time: 40 minutes

Servings: 8

Ingredients:

- tablespoon Greek seasoning
- A pinch of salt and black pepper
- tablespoon capers
- tablespoon olive oil
- 4 spring onions, chopped
- garlic clove, minced
- teaspoons basil, chopped
- teaspoons oregano, chopped
- cup brown rice
- cups chicken stock
- ¼ cup kalamata olives, pitted and sliced
- ¼ cup sun-dried tomatoes, chopped
- tablespoons lemon juice
- teaspoons parsley, chopped
- pound chicken breast boneless, skinless and cubed

Directions:

1. Heat a saucepan with the oil over medium heat, add the chicken and brown for 2-3 minutes.
2. Add Greek seasoning, salt, pepper and the garlic, stir and cook for 3 minutes more.
3. Add the capers, spring onions, basil, oregano, rice, stock, olives, tomatoes, and lemon juice, stir, bring to a boil and simmer for 30 minutes.
4. Add the parsley, stir, ladle the soup into bowls and serve.

Nutrition Values: Calories 271, Fat 5g, Fiber 1g, Carbs 13g, Protein 16g

HEALTHY MEDITERRANEAN CHICKEN

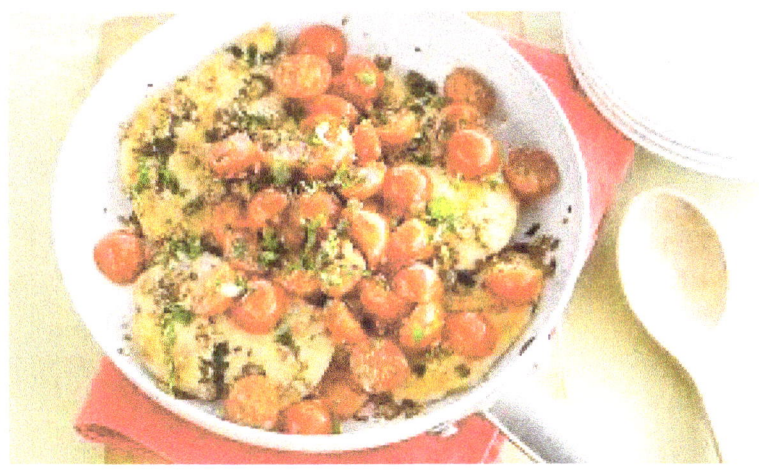

PREPARATION TIME: 5 MINUTES
COOKING TIME: 6 HOURS AND 10 MINUTES
SERVINGS: 6

. . .

Ingredients:

- 2 pounds chicken breasts, boneless and skinless
- 28 ounces canned tomatoes, chopped
- 28 ounces canned artichoke hearts, drained
- ½ cups chicken stock yellow onion, chopped
- ¼ cup white wine vinegar
- ½ cup kalamata olives, pitted and chopped
- tablespoon curry powder
- teaspoons thyme
- teaspoons basil
- Salt and black pepper to taste
- ¼ cup parsley, chopped

Directions:

1. Put chicken breasts in a slow cooker.
2. Add tomatoes, artichoke hearts, onion and olives and stir.
3. Add stock, vinegar, curry powder, thyme, basil, salt and black pepper to taste.
4. Cover and cook on Low for 6 hours. Uncover, add more salt and pepper if needed, add parsley and stir gently.

Nutrition Values: Calories 342, Fat 3g, Fiber 3g, Carbs 5g, Protein 4g

MUSHROOM AND CHICKEN BOWL

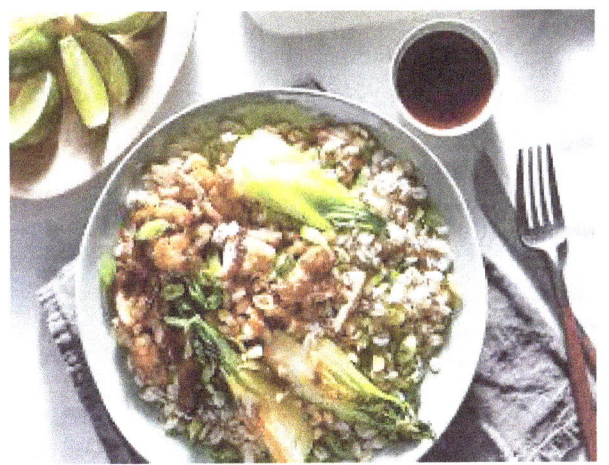

Preparation time: 10 minutes
Cooking time: 25 minutes
Servings: 4

Ingredients

- 1 and ½ cups unsweetened coconut milk
- 1 pound chicken thigh, skinless
- 3-4 garlic cloves, crushed
- ½ an onion, finely diced
- 2-inch knob ginger, minced
- 1 cup mushrooms, sliced
- 4 ounces baby spinach
- ½ teaspoon of cayenne pepper
- ½ teaspoon turmeric
- 1 teaspoon salt
- 1 teaspoon Garam Masala
- ¼ cup cilantro, chopped

Directions

1. Add the listed ingredients to your Ninja Foodi
2. Lock lid and cook on HIGH pressure for 15 minutes
3. Release pressure naturally over 10 minutes
4. Remove chicken and roughly puree the veggies using an immersion blender
5. Shred chicken and add it back to the pot. Add cream and stir. Serve and enjoy!

Nutrition Values: Calories 200, Fat 15g, Fiber 3g, Carbs 10g, Protein 33g

CHICKEN AND BROCCOLI PLATTER

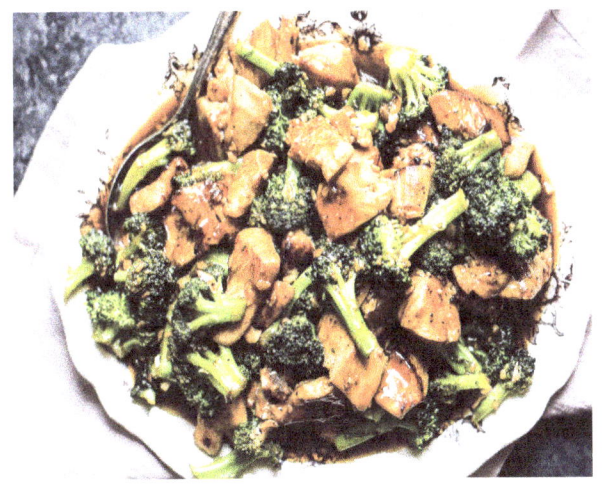

Preparation time: 10 minutes
Cooking time: 20 minutes
Servings: 4

. . .

Ingredients

- 1 tablespoon olive oil
- 1 tablespoon butter
- 2 large chicken breasts, boneless
- ½ cup onion, chopped
- 14 ounces chicken broth
- ½ teaspoon salt
- ½ teaspoon pepper
- 1/8 teaspoon red pepper flakes
- 1 tablespoon parsley
- 1 tablespoon arrowroot
- 2 tablespoons water
- 4 ounces light cream cheese, cubed
- 1 cup cheddar cheese, shredded
- 3 cups steamed broccoli, chopped

Directions

1. Season the chicken breast with pepper and salt
2. Set your Ninja Foodi to Saute mode and add butter and vegetable oil
3. Allow it to melt and transfer the seasoned chicken to the pot. Allow it to brown
4. Remove the chicken and add the onions to the pot, Saute them for 5 minutes
5. Add chicken broth, pepper, red pepper and salt, parsley. Add the browned breast
6. Lock up the lid and cook for about 5 minutes at high pressure
7. Once done, quick release the pressure. Remove the chicken and shred it up into small portions
8. Take a bowl and add 2 tablespoons of water and dissolve cornstarch \
9. Select the simmer mode and add the mixture to the Ninja Foodi

10. Toss in the cubed and shredded cheese. Stir completely until everything is melted
11. Toss in the diced chicken again and the steamed broccoli and cook for 5 minutes
12. Once done, sever with white rice and shredded cheese as garnish

Nutrition Values: Calories 230, Fat 12g, Fiber 12g, Carbs 34g, Protein 13g

DARING SALTED BAKED CHICKEN

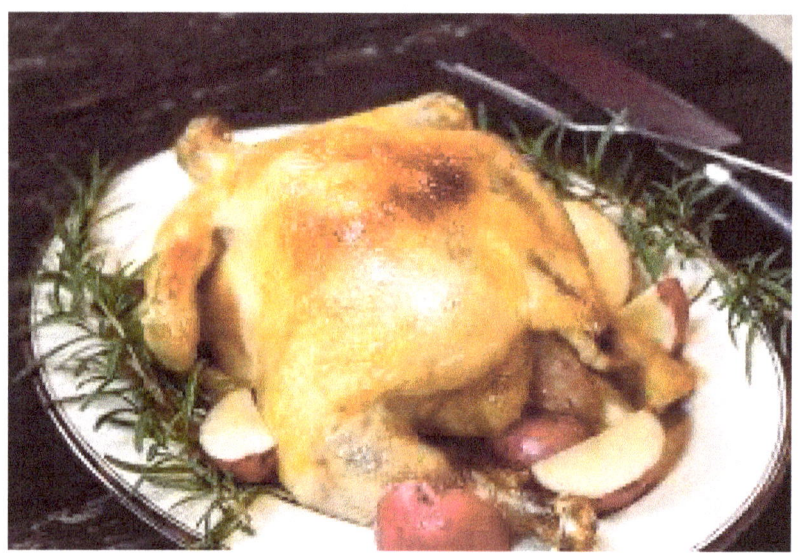

PREPARATION TIME: 10 MINUTES
COOKING TIME: 26 MINUTES
SERVINGS: 6

· · ·

Ingredients

- 2 teaspoons ginger, minced
- 1 and ¼ teaspoons salt
- ¼ teaspoons five spice powder
- Dash of white pepper
- 5-6 chicken legs

Directions

1. Season the chicken legs by placing them in a large mixing bowl
2. Pour 2 teaspoon of ginger, 1 and a ¼ teaspoon of kosher salt, ¼ teaspoon of five spice powder and mix
3. Transfer them to a parchment paper
4. Wrap up tightly and place them to a shallow dish
5. Place a steamer rack in your Ninja Foodi and add 1 cup of water
6. Place the chicken dish onto the rack
7. Lock up the lid and cook on HIGH pressure for 18-26 minutes
8. Release the pressure naturally
9. Open the lid and unwrap the paper
10. Pour the juice into a small bowl
11. Transfer the chicken on a wire rack and broil for a while
12. Serve immediately with the cooking liquid used as a dipping sauce

Nutrition Values: Calories 145, Fat 4g, Fiber 3g, Carbs 11g, Protein 4g

WORTHY GHEE-LICIOUS CHICKEN

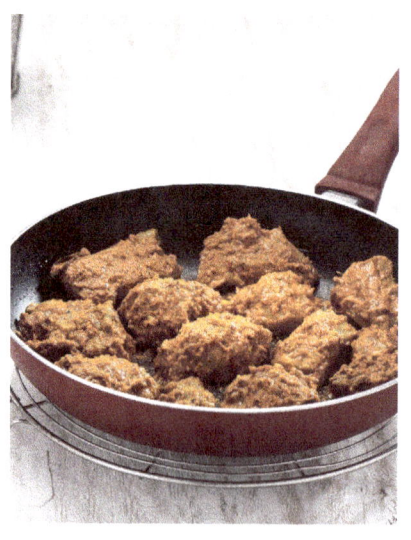

Preparation time: 5 minutes
Cooking time: 10 minutes
Servings: 6

Ingredients

- 2-3 pounds boneless chicken thigh
- 1 tablespoon ghee
- 1 and a ½ large onion, chopped
- 3 and ½ teaspoons salt
- 2 teaspoons garlic powder
- 2 teaspoons ginger powder
- 2 heaping teaspoons turmeric
- 1 and ½ teaspoon cayenne powder
- 1 and ½ cup stewed tomatoes
- 1 cup stewed tomatoes
- 2 cans of coconut milk
- 2 heaping teaspoons Garam masala
- ½ cup almond, sliced
- ½ cup cilantro

Directions

1. Set your Ninja Foodi to Saute mode and add ghee, allow it to melt
2. Add 2 teaspoon of salt alongside onion and cook well
3. Add ginger, garlic, turmeric, paprika, cayenne pepper and mix well
4. Add your canned tomatoes alongside coconut milk and mix
5. Add chicken and give it a nice stir
6. Lock up the lid and cook on HIGH pressure for about 8 minutes
7. Once done, pour coconut cream, tomato paste, and Garam Masala
8. Garnish with some cilantro and serve with a sprinkle of sliced up almonds. Enjoy!

Nutrition Values: Calories 230, Fat 12g, Fiber 12g, Carbs 34g, Protein 13g

CHICKEN KORMA

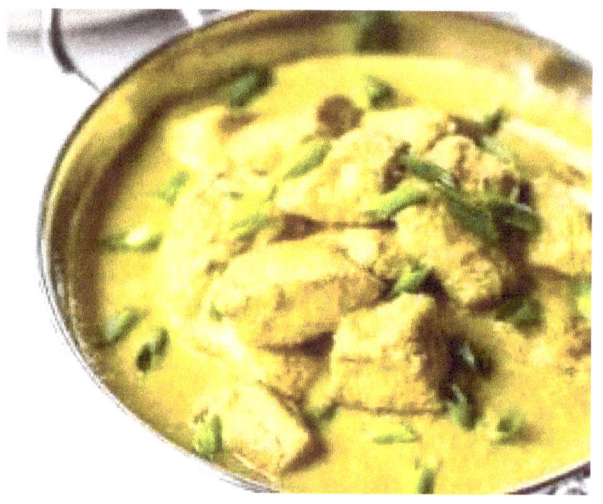

Preparation time: 5 minutes
Cooking time: 10 minutes
Servings: 6

. . .

Ingredients

- 1 pound of chicken
- For Sauce
- 1 ounce of cashews
- 1 small chopped onion
- ½ a cup of diced tomatoes
- ½ of green Serrano pepper
- 5 cloves of garlic
- 1 teaspoon of minced ginger
- 1 teaspoon of turmeric
- 1 teaspoon of Garam masala
- 1 teaspoon of cumin-coriander powder
- ½ a teaspoon of cayenne pepper
- ½ a cup of water

For topping

- 1 teaspoon of Garam masala
- ½ a cup of coconut milk
- ¼ cup of chopped cilantro

Directions

1. Add the sauce ingredients to a blender and blend them well
2. Pour the sauce to your Ninja Foodi. Place the chicken on top
3. Lock up the lid and cook on HIGH pressure for 10 minutes
4. Release the pressure naturally. Take the chicken out and cut into bite-sized portions
5. Add coconut milk, Garam masala to the pot
6. Transfer the chicken back and garnish with cilantro. Enjoy!

Nutrition Values: Calories 145, Fat 4g, Fiber 3g, Carbs 11g, Protein 4g

TURKEY WITH GARLIC SAUCE

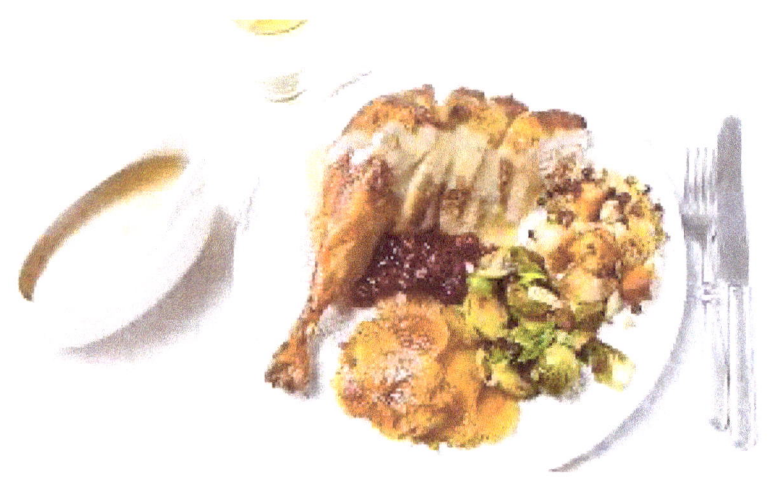

Preparation time: 5 minutes
Cooking time: 1 hour
Servings: 6

Ingredients

- 5 large onions, thinly sliced
- 4 garlic cloves, minced
- ¼ cup white wine vinegar
- ½ teaspoon salt
- ¼ teaspoon ground black pepper
- ¼ teaspoon cayenne pepper
- 4 large skinless turkey thighs

Directions

1. Gently lay the garlic and onions into the bottom of your Ninja Foodi
2. Pour in some wine with a sprinkle of salt, cayenne pepper, and black pepper.
3. Add turkey thighs and cover it up. Let it cook SLOW COOKER MODE (low) for about 1 hour.
4. Remove the turkey from the crock pot and clean up the flesh from the bones.
5. Keep the lid open and keep cooking until the liquid has completely evaporated, making sure to stir from time to time. Return the turkey to the pot.
6. Nestle the turkey into the mix. Serve hot. Enjoy!

Nutrition Values: Calories 200, Fat 15g, Fiber 3g, Carbs 10g, Protein 33g

Part Four
SNACKS & DESSERTS

HEALTHY COCONUT BLUEBERRY BALLS

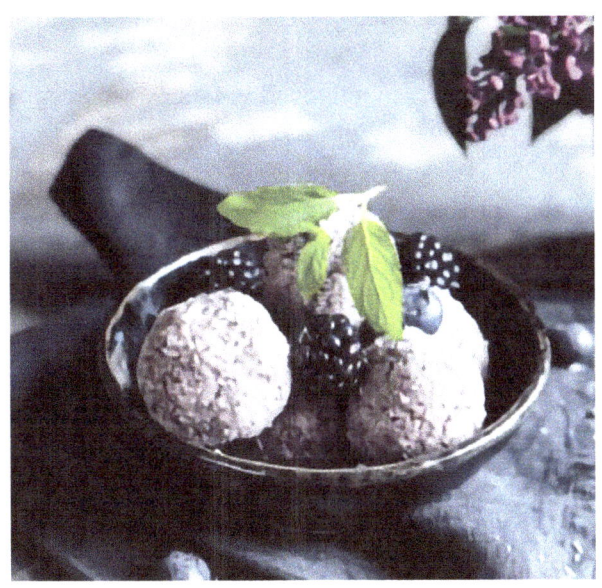

Preparation Time: 10 minutes
Cooking Time: 10 minutes
Serve: 12

Ingredients:

- ¼ cup flaked coconut
- ¼ cup blueberries
- ½ tsp vanilla
- ¼ cup honey
- ½ cup creamy almond butter
- ¼ tsp cinnamon
- 1 ½ tbsp chia seeds
- ¼ cup flaxseed meal
- 1 cup rolled oats, gluten-free

Directions:

1. In a large bowl, add oats, cinnamon, chia seeds, and flaxseed meal and mix well.
2. Add almond butter in microwave-safe bowl and microwave for 30 seconds. Stir until smooth.
3. Add vanilla and honey in melted almond butter and stir well.
4. Pour almond butter mixture over oat mixture and stir to combine.
5. Add coconut and blueberries and stir well.
6. Make small balls from oat mixture and place onto the baking tray and place in the refrigerator for 1 hour.
7. Serve and enjoy.

Nutritional Value: Calories 129, Fat 7.4g, Carbohydrates 14.1g, Sugar 7g, Protein 4 g, Cholesterol 0 mg

CRUNCHY ROASTED CHICKPEAS

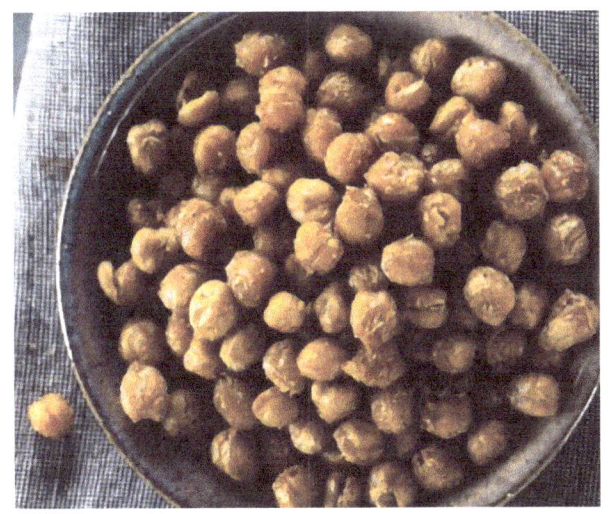

Preparation Time: 10 minutes
Cooking Time: 25 minutes
Serve: 4

. . .

Ingredients:

- 15 oz can chickpeas, drained, rinsed and pat dry
- ¼ tsp paprika
- 1 tbsp olive oil
- ¼ tsp pepper
- Pinch of salt

Directions:

1. Preheat the oven to 450 F.
2. Spray a baking tray with cooking spray and set aside.
3. In a large bowl, toss chickpeas with olive oil and spread chickpeas onto the prepared baking tray.
4. Roast chickpeas in preheated oven for 25 minutes. Shake after every 10 minutes.
5. Once chickpeas are done then immediately toss with paprika, pepper, and salt.
6. Serve and enjoy.

Nutritional Value: Calories 157, Fat 4.7g, Carbohydrates 24.2g, Sugar 0g, Protein 5.3g, Cholesterol 0mg

TASTY ZUCCHINI CHIPS

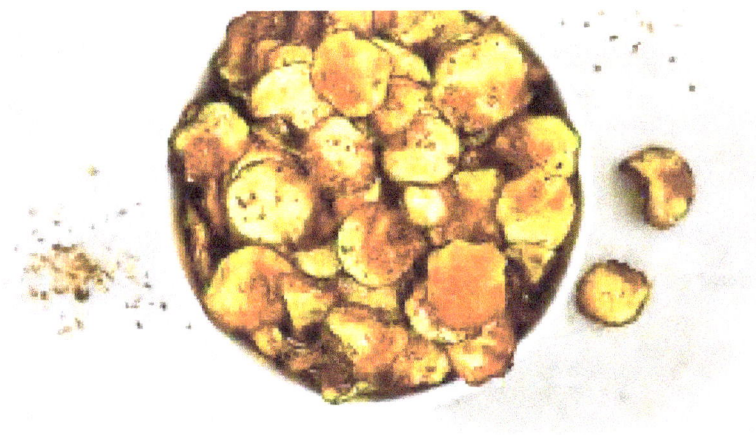

Preparation Time: 10 minutes
Cooking Time: 15 minutes
Serve: 8

Ingredients:

- 2 medium zucchini, sliced 4mm thick
- ½ tsp paprika
- ¼ tsp garlic powder
- ¾ cup parmesan cheese, grated
- 4 tbsp olive oil
- ¼ tsp pepper
- Pinch of salt

Directions:

1. Preheat the oven to 375 F.
2. Spray a baking tray with cooking spray and set aside.
3. In a bowl, combine the oil, garlic powder, paprika, pepper, and salt.
4. Add sliced zucchini and toss to coat.
5. Arrange zucchini slices onto the prepared baking tray and sprinkle grated cheese on top.
6. Bake in preheated oven for 15 minutes or until lightly golden brown.
7. Serve and enjoy.

Nutritional Value: Calories 110, Fat 9.8g, Carbohydrates 2.2g, Sugar 0.9g, Protein 4.4g, Cholesterol 7mg

ROASTED GREEN BEANS

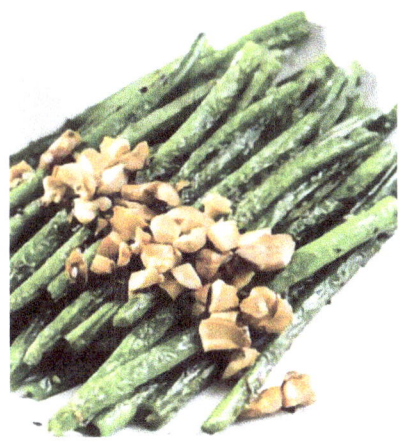

Preparation Time: 10 minutes
Cooking Time: 15 minutes
Serve: 4

. . .

Ingredients:

- 1 lb green beans
- 4 tbsp parmesan cheese
- 2 tbsp olive oil
- ¼ tsp garlic powder
- Pinch of salt

Directions:

1. Preheat the oven to 400 F.
2. Add green beans in a large bowl.
3. Add remaining ingredients on top of green beans and toss to coat.
4. Spread green beans onto the baking tray and roast in preheated oven for 15 minutes. Stir halfway through.
5. Serve and enjoy.

Nutritional Value: Calories 101, Fat 7.5g, Carbohydrates 8.3g, Sugar 1.6g, Protein 2.6g, Cholesterol 1mg

SAVORY PISTACHIO BALLS

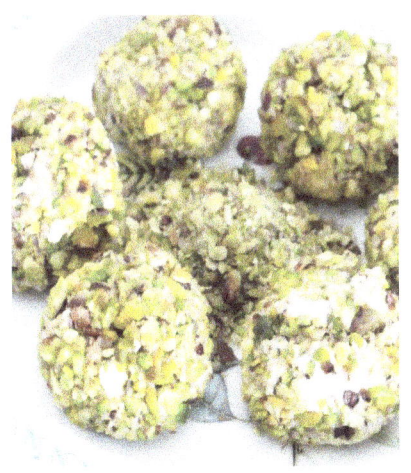

Preparation Time: 10 minutes
Cooking Time: 5 minutes
Serve: 16

. . .

Ingredients:

- ½ cup pistachios, unsalted
- 1 cup dates, pitted
- ½ tsp ground fennel seeds
- ½ cup raisins
- Pinch of pepper

Directions:

1. Add all ingredients into the food processor and process until well combined.
2. Make small balls and place onto the baking tray and place in the refrigerator for 1 hour.
3. Serve and enjoy.

Nutritional Value: Calories 55, Fat 0.9g, Carbohydrates 12.5g, Sugar 9.9g, Protein 0.8g, Cholesterol 0mg

ROASTED ALMONDS

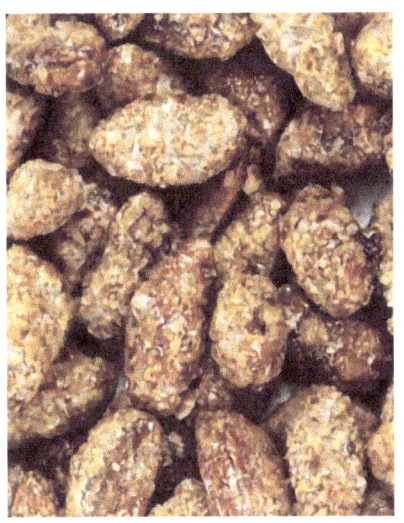

Preparation Time: 10 minutes
Cooking Time: 20 minutes
Serve: 12

• • •

Ingredients:

- 2 ½ cups almonds
- ¼ tsp cayenne
- ¼ tsp ground coriander
- ¼ tsp cumin
- ¼ tsp chili powder
- 1 tbsp fresh rosemary, chopped
- 1 tbsp olive oil
- 2 ½ tbsp maple syrup
- Pinch of salt

Directions:

1. Preheat the oven to 325 F.
2. Spray a baking tray with cooking spray and set aside.
3. In a mixing bowl, whisk together oil, cayenne, coriander, cumin, chili powder, rosemary, maple syrup, and salt.
4. Add almond and stir to coat.
5. Spread almonds onto the prepared baking tray.
6. Roast almonds in preheated oven for 20 minutes. Stir halfway through.
7. Serve and enjoy.

Nutritional Value: Calories 137, Fat 11.2g, Carbohydrates 7.3g, Sugar 3.3g, Protein 4.2g, Cholesterol 0mg

BANANA STRAWBERRY POPSICLES

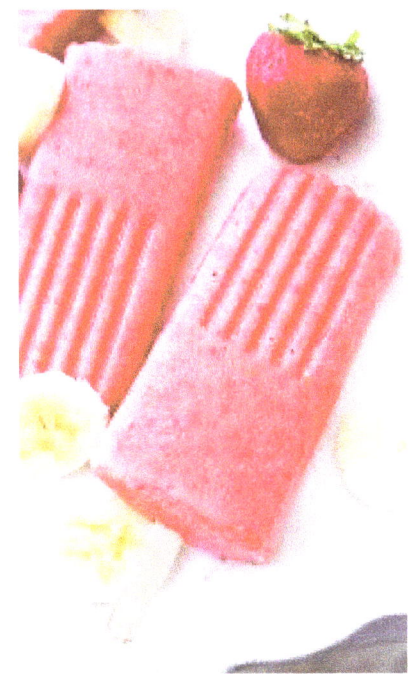

Preparation Time: 5 minutes

Cooking Time: 0 minutes
Serve: 8

Ingredients:

- ½ cup Greek yogurt
- 1 banana, peeled and sliced
- 1 ¼ cup fresh strawberries
- ¼ cup of water

Directions:

1. Add all ingredients into the blender and blend until smooth.
2. Pour blended mixture into the popsicles molds and place in the refrigerator for 4 hours or until set.
3. Serve and enjoy.

Nutritional Value: Calories 31, Fat 0. g, Carbohydrates 6.2g, Sugar 4g, Protein 1.2g ,Cholesterol 1mg

CHOCOLATE MATCHA BALLS

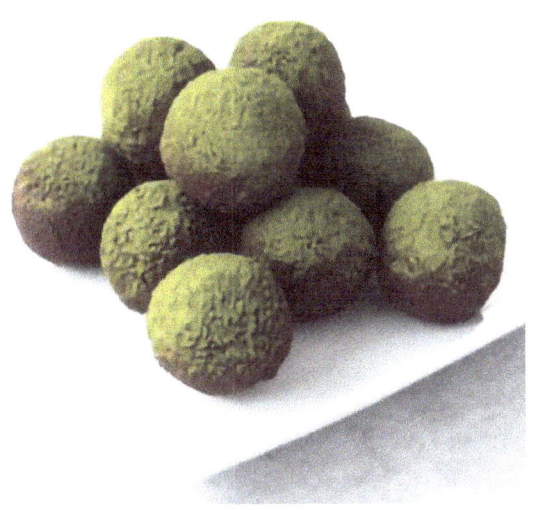

Preparation Time: 10 minutes
Cooking Time: 5 minutes

Serve: 15

Ingredients:

- 2 tbsp unsweetened cocoa powder
- 3 tbsp oats, gluten-free
- ½ cup pine nuts
- ½ cup almonds
- 1 cup dates, pitted
- 2 tbsp matcha powder

Directions:

1. Add oats, pine nuts, almonds, and dates into a food processor and process until well combined.
2. Place matcha powder in a small dish.
3. Make small balls from mixture and coat with matcha powder.
4. Enjoy or store in refrigerator until ready to eat.

Nutritional Value: Calories 88, Fat 4.9g, Carbohydrates 11.3g, Sugar 7.8g, Protein 1.9g, Cholesterol 0mg

CHIA ALMOND BUTTER PUDDING

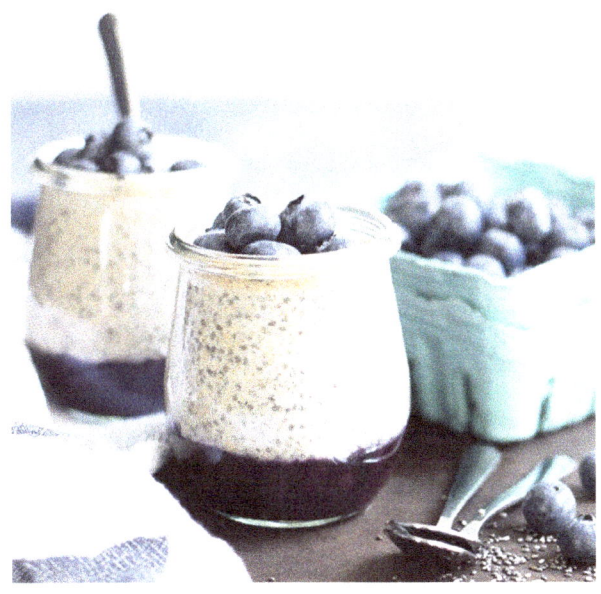

Preparation Time: 5 minutes
Cooking Time: 5 minutes
Serve: 1

Ingredients:

- ¼ cup chia seeds
- 1 cup unsweetened almond milk
- 1 ½ tbsp maple syrup
- 2 ½ tbsp almond butter

Directions:

1. Add almond milk, maple syrup, and almond butter in a bowl and stir well.
2. Add chia seeds and stir to mix.
3. Pour pudding mixture into the Mason jar and place in the refrigerator for overnight.
4. Serve and enjoy.

Nutritional Value: Calories 354, Fat 21.3g, Carbohydrates 31.1g, Sugar 18.9g, Protein 11.2g, Cholesterol 0mg

REFRESHING STRAWBERRY POPSICLES

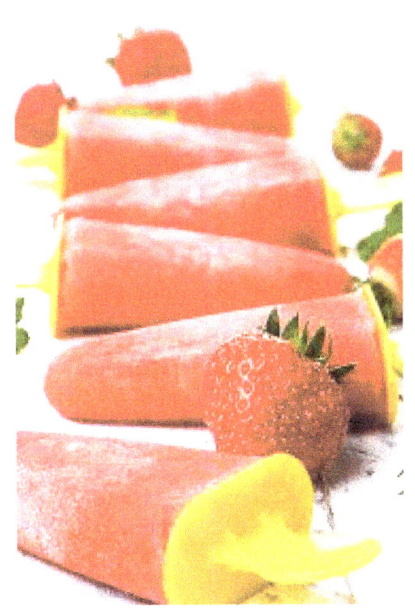

Preparation Time: 5 minutes
Cooking Time: 5 minutes

Serve: 8

Ingredients:

- ½ cup almond milk
- 2 ½ cup fresh strawberries

Directions:

1. Add strawberries and almond milk into the blender and blend until smooth.
2. Pour strawberry mixture into popsicles molds and place in the refrigerator for 4 hours or until set.
3. Serve and enjoy.

Nutritional Value: Calories 49, Fat 3.7g, Carbohydrates 4.3g, Sugar 2.7g, Protein 0.6g, Cholesterol 0mg

DARK CHOCOLATE MOUSSE

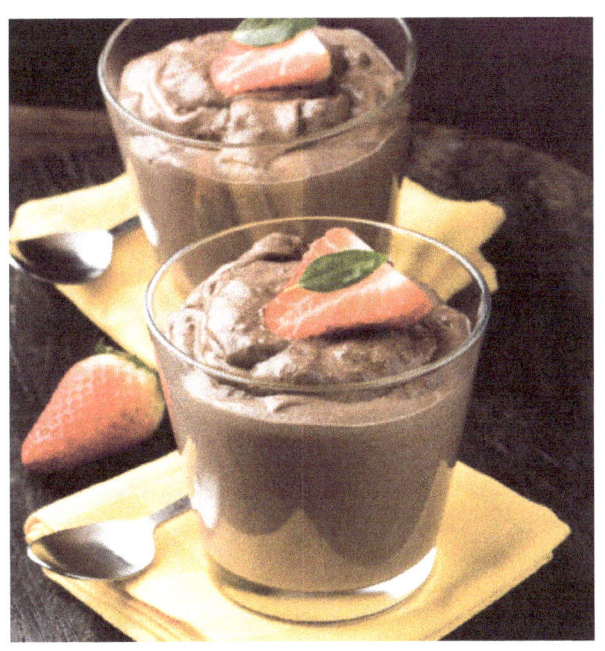

Preparation Time: 10 minutes
Cooking Time: 10 minutes
Serve: 4

Ingredients:

- 3.5 oz unsweetened dark chocolate, grated
- ½ tsp vanilla
- 1 tbsp honey
- 2 cups Greek yogurt
- ¾ cup unsweetened almond milk

Directions:

1. Add chocolate and almond milk in a saucepan and heat over medium heat until just chocolate melted. Do not boil.
2. Once the chocolate and almond milk combined then add vanilla and honey and stir well.
3. Add yogurt in a large mixing bowl.
4. Pour chocolate mixture on top of yogurt and mix until well combined.
5. Pour chocolate yogurt mixture into the serving bowls and place in refrigerator for 2 hours.
6. Top with fresh raspberries and serve.

Nutritional Value: Calories 278, Fat 15.4g, Carbohydrates 20g, Sugar 13g, Protein 10.5g, Cholesterol 7mg

WARM & SOFT BAKED PEARS

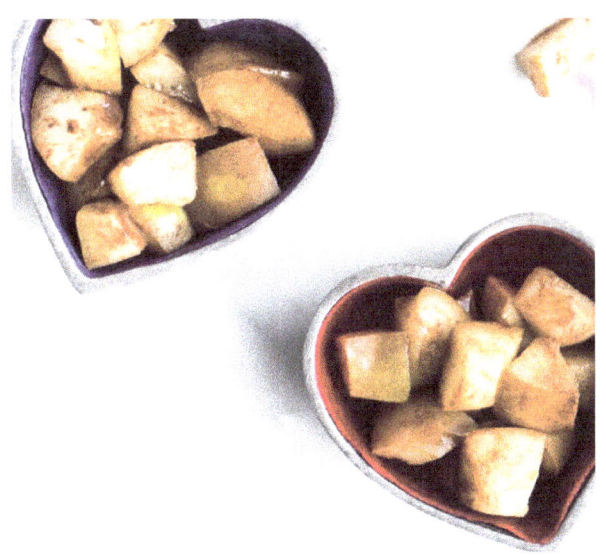

Preparation Time: 10 minutes
Cooking Time: 25 minutes
Serve: 4

. . .

Ingredients:

- 4 pears, cut in half and core
- ½ tsp vanilla
- ¼ tsp cinnamon
- ½ cup maple syrup

Directions:

1. Preheat the oven to 375 F.
2. Spray a baking tray with cooking spray.
3. Arrange pears, cut side up on a prepared baking tray and sprinkle with cinnamon.
4. In a small bowl, whisk vanilla and maple syrup and drizzle over pears.
5. Bake pears in preheated oven for 25 minutes.
6. Serve and enjoy.

Nutritional Value: Calories 226, Fat 0.4g, Carbohydrates 58.4g, Sugar 43.9g, Protein 0.8g, Cholesterol 0mg

HEALTHY & QUICK ENERGY BITES

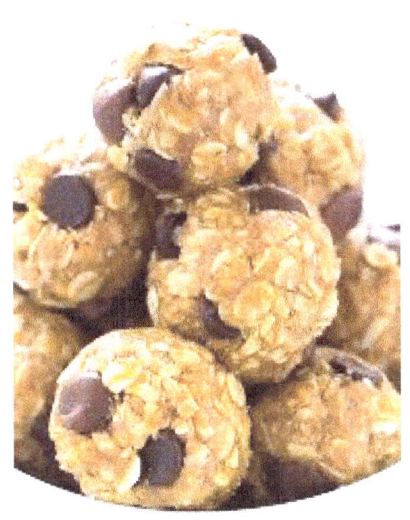

Preparation Time: 10 minutes
Cooking Time: 0 minutes
Serve: 20

Ingredients:

- 2 cups cashew nuts
- ¼ tsp cinnamon
- 1 tsp lemon zest
- 4 tbsp dates, chopped
- 1/3 cup unsweetened shredded coconut
- ¾ cup dried apricots

Directions:

1. Line baking tray with parchment paper and set aside.
2. Add all ingredients in a food processor and process until the mixture is crumbly and well combined.
3. Make small balls from mixture and place on a prepared baking tray.
4. Place in refrigerator for 1 hour.
5. Serve and enjoy.

Nutritional Value: Calories 100, Fat 7.5g, Carbohydrates 7.2g, Sugar 2.8g, Protein 2.4g, Cholesterol 0mg

CREAMY YOGURT BANANA BOWLS

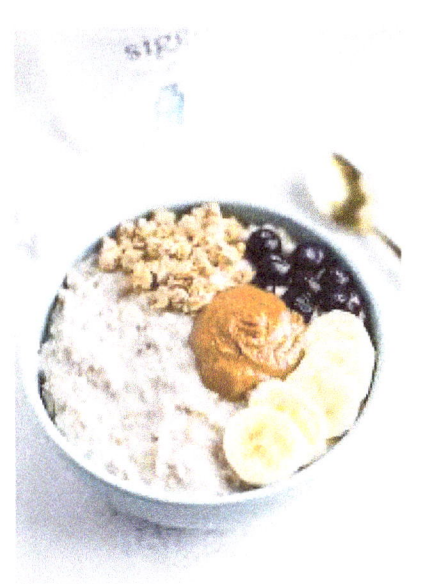

Preparation Time: 10 minutes
Cooking Time: 0 minutes

Serve: 4

Ingredients:

- 2 bananas, sliced
- ½ tsp ground nutmeg
- 3 tbsp flaxseed meal
- ¼ cup creamy peanut butter
- 4 cups Greek yogurt

Directions:

1. Divide Greek yogurt between 4 serving bowls and top with sliced bananas.
2. Add peanut butter in microwave-safe bowl and microwave for 30 seconds.
3. Drizzle 1 tablespoon of melted peanut butter on each bowl on top of the sliced bananas.
4. Sprinkle cinnamon and flax meal on top and serve.

Nutritional Value: Calories 351, Fat 13.1g, Carbohydrates 35.6g, Sugar 26.1g, Protein 19.6g, Cholesterol 15mg

CHOCOLATE MOUSSE

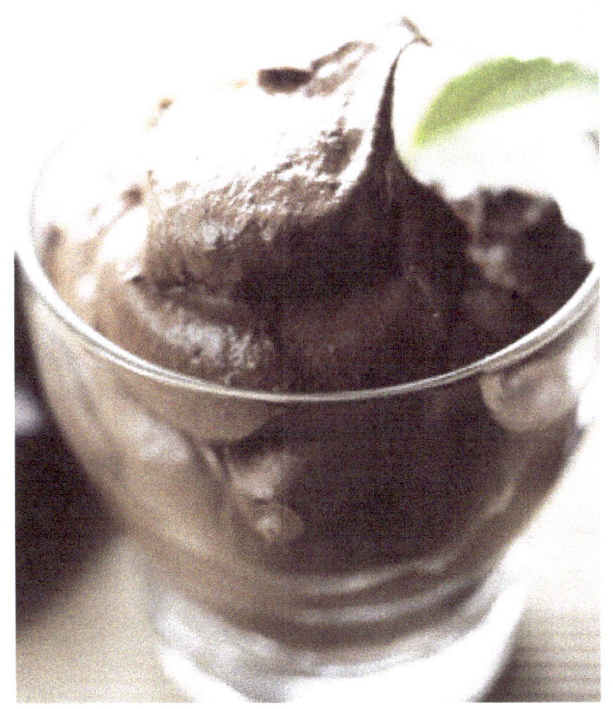

Preparation Time: 10 minutes
Cooking Time: 6 minutes
Serve: 5

Ingredients:

- 4 egg yolks
- ½ tsp vanilla
- ½ cup unsweetened almond milk
- 1 cup whipping cream
- ¼ cup cocoa powder
- ¼ cup water
- ½ cup Swerve
- 1/8 tsp salt

Directions:

1. Add egg yolks to a large bowl and whisk until well beaten.
2. In a saucepan, add swerve, cocoa powder, and water and whisk until well combined.
3. Add almond milk and cream to the saucepan and whisk until well mix.
4. Once saucepan mixtures are heated up then turn off the heat.
5. Add vanilla and salt and stir well.
6. Add a tablespoon of chocolate mixture into the eggs and whisk until well combined.
7. Slowly pour remaining chocolate to the eggs and whisk until well combined.
8. Pour batter into the ramekins.
9. Pour 1 ½ cups of water into the instant pot then place a trivet in the pot.
10. Place ramekins on a trivet.
11. Seal pot with lid and select manual and set timer for 6 minutes.

12. Release pressure using quick release method than open the lid.
13. Carefully remove ramekins from the instant pot and let them cool completely.
14. Serve and enjoy.

Nutrition Values: Calories 128, Fat 11.9g, Carbohydrates 4g, Sugar 0.2g, Protein 3.6g, Cholesterol 194mg

CARROT SPREAD

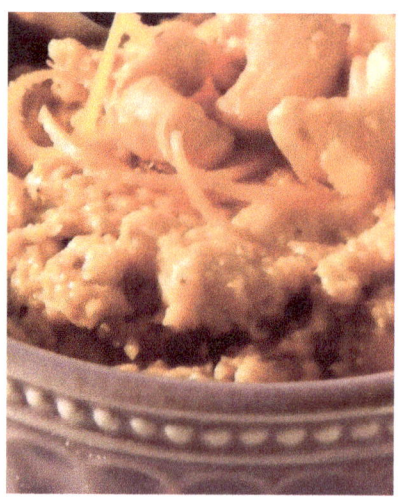

Preparation time: 10 minutes
Cooking time: 10 minutes
Serves: 4

· · ·

Ingredients:
- ¼ cup veggie stock
- A pinch of salt and black pepper
- 1 teaspoon onion powder
- ½ teaspoon garlic powder
- ½ teaspoon oregano, dried
- 1 pound carrots, sliced
- ½ cup coconut cream

Directions:

1. In your instant pot, combine all the ingredients except the cream, put the lid on and cook on High for 10 minutes.
2. Release the pressure naturally for 10 minutes, transfer the carrots mix to food processor, add the cream, pulse well, divide into bowls and serve cold.

Nutrition Values: Calories 124, Fat 1g, Fiber 2g, Carbs 5g, Protein 8g

CHICKEN WINGS PLATTER

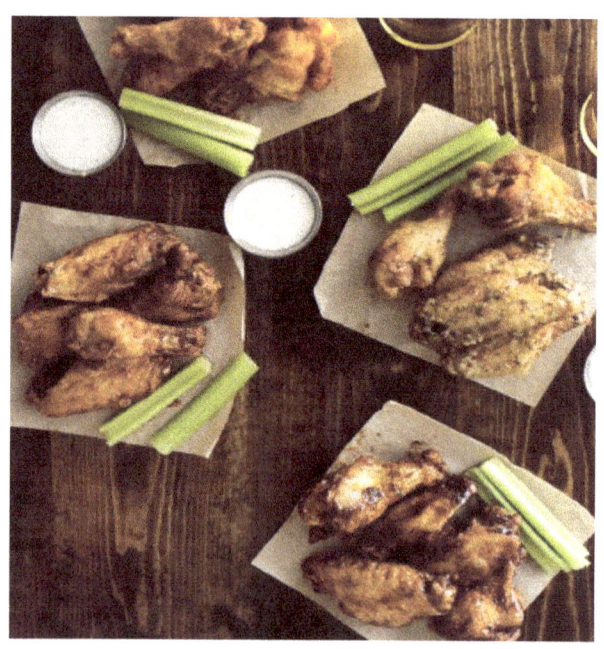

Preparation time: 10 minutes
Cooking time: 20 minutes
Serves: 4

Ingredients:
- 2 pounds chicken wings
- ½ cup tomato sauce
- A pinch of salt and black pepper
- 1 teaspoon smoked paprika
- 1 tablespoon cilantro, chopped
- 1 tablespoon chives, chopped

Directions:
1. In your instant pot, combine the chicken wings with the sauce and the rest of the ingredients, stir, put the lid on and cook on High for 20 minutes.
2. Release the pressure naturally for 10 minutes, arrange the chicken wings on a platter and serve as an appetizer.

Nutrition Values: Calories 203, Fat 13g, Fiber 3g, Carbs 5g, Protein 8g

STUFFED CHICKEN

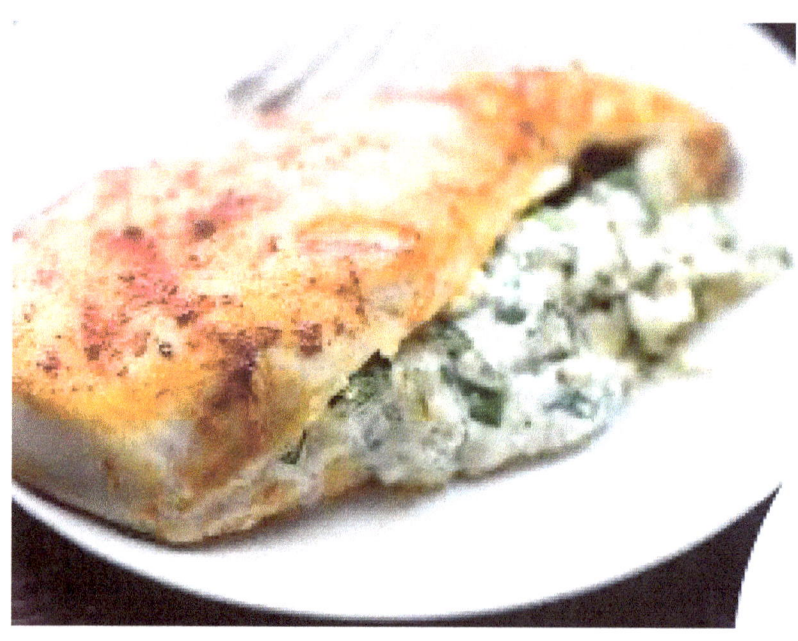

Preparation time: 10 minutes
Cooking time: 30 minutes

Serves: 4

Ingredients:
- 4 chicken breasts, skinless, boneless and butterflied
- 1 ounce spring onions, chopped
- ½ pound white mushrooms, sliced
- 1 teaspoon hot paprika
- A pinch of salt and black pepper
- 1 cup tomato sauce

Directions:

1. Flatten chicken breasts with a meat mallet and place them on a plate.
2. In a bowl, mix the spring onions with the mushrooms, paprika, salt and pepper and stir well.
3. Divide this on each chicken breast half, roll them and secure with a toothpick.
4. Add the tomato sauce in the instant pot, put the chicken rolls inside as well. put the lid on and cook on High for 30 minutes.
5. Release the pressure naturally for 10 minutes, arrange the stuffed chicken breasts on a platter and serve.

Nutrition Values: Calories 221, Fat 12g, Fiber 3g, Carbs 6g, Protein 11g

CINNAMON BABY BACK RIBS PLATTER

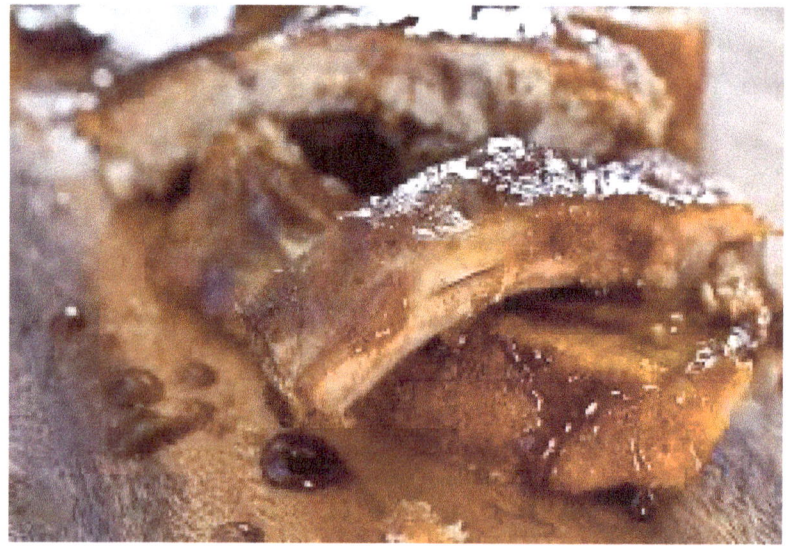

Preparation time: 10 minutes
Cooking time: 40 minutes
Serves: 2

. . .

Ingredients:
- 1 rack baby back ribs
- 2 teaspoons smoked paprika
- 2 teaspoon chili powder
- A pinch of salt and black pepper
- 1 teaspoon garlic powder
- 1 teaspoon onion powder
- 1 teaspoon cinnamon powder
- ½ teaspoon cumin seeds
- A pinch of cayenne pepper
- 1 cup tomato sauce
- 3 garlic cloves, minced

Directions:

1. In your instant pot, combine the baby back ribs with the rest of the ingredients, put the lid on and cook on High for 30 minutes.
2. Release the pressure naturally for 10 minutes, arrange the ribs on a platter and serve as an appetizer.

Nutrition Values: Calories 222, Fat 12g, Fiber 4g, Carbs 6g, Protein 14g

BUTTERY CARROT STICKS

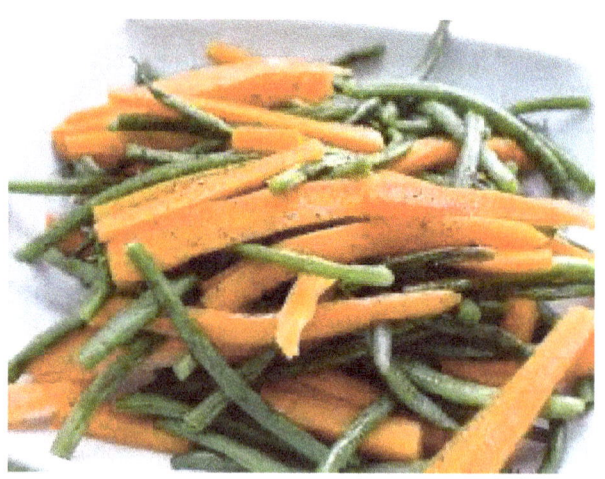

Preparation time: 10 minutes
Cooking time: 15 minutes
Serves: 4

. . .

Ingredients:
- 1 pound carrot, cut into sticks
- 4 garlic cloves, minced
- ¼ cup chicken stock
- 1 teaspoon rosemary, chopped
- A pinch of salt and black pepper
- 2 tablespoons olive oil
- 2 tablespoons ghee, melted

Directions:

1. Set the instant pot on Sauté mode, add the oil and the ghee, heat them up, add the garlic and brown for 1 minute.

2. Add the rest of the ingredients, put the lid on and cook on High for 14 minutes.

3. Release the pressure naturally for 10 minutes, arrange the carrot sticks on a platter and serve.

Nutrition Values: Calories 142, Fat 4g, Fiber 2g, Carbs 5g, Protein 7g

CAJUN WALNUTS AND OLIVES BOWLS

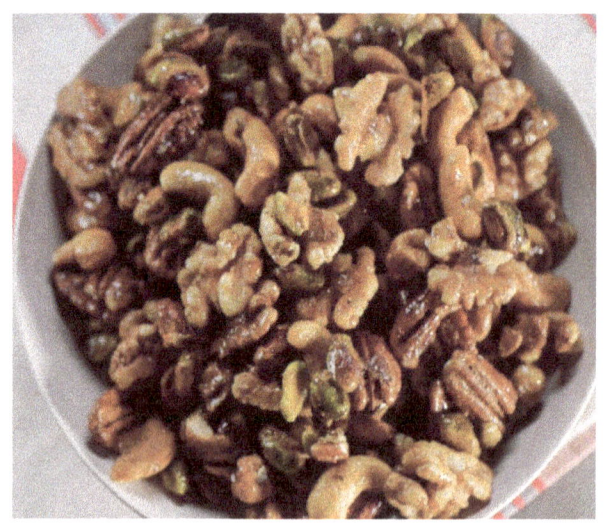

Preparation time: 10 minutes
Cooking time: 10 minutes
Serves: 2

Ingredients:
- ½ pound walnuts, chopped
- A pinch of salt and black pepper
- 1 and ½ cups black olives, pitted
- ½ tablespoon Cajun seasoning
- 2 garlic cloves, minced
- 1 red chili pepper, chopped
- ¼ cup veggie stock
- 2 tablespoon tomato puree

Directions:

1. In your instant pot, combine the walnuts with the olives and the rest of the ingredients, put the lid on and cook on High 10 minutes.

2. Release the pressure fast for 5 minutes, divide the mix into small bowls and serve as an appetizer.

Nutrition Values: Calories 105, Fat 1g, Fiber 1g, Carbs 4g, Protein 7g

MANGO SALSA

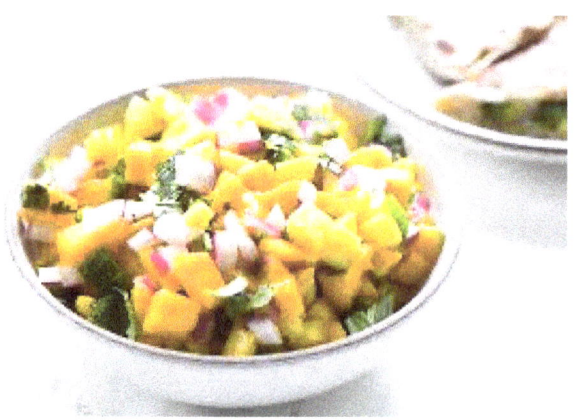

Preparation time: 10 minutes
Cooking time: 10 minutes
Serves: 2

. . .

Ingredients:
- 2 mangoes, peeled and cubed
- ½ tablespoon sweet paprika
- 2 garlic cloves, minced
- 2 tablespoons cilantro, chopped
- 1 tablespoon spring onions, chopped
- 1 cup cherry tomatoes, cubed
- 1 cup avocado, peeled, pitted and cubed
- A pinch of salt and black pepper
- 1 tablespoon olive oil
- ¼ cup tomato puree
- ½ cup kalamata olives, pitted and sliced

Directions:

1. In your instant pot, combine the mangoes with the paprika and the rest of the ingredients except the cilantro, put the lid on and cook on High for 5 minutes.

2. Release the pressure fast for 5 minutes, divide the mix into small bowls, sprinkle the cilantro on top and serve.

Nutrition Values: Calories 123, Fat 4g, Fiber 1g, Carbs 3g, Protein 5g

HOT ASPARAGUS STICKS

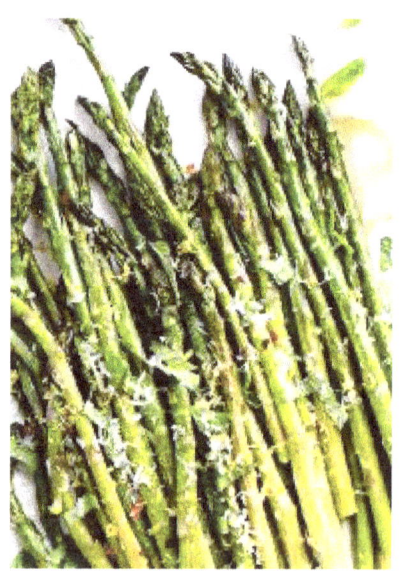

Preparation time: 10 minutes
Cooking time: 10 minutes
Serves: 2

. . .

Ingredients:
- 1 and ½ pounds asparagus, trimmed
- 2 tablespoons olive oil
- 2 tablespoons cayenne pepper sauce
- A pinch of salt and black pepper
- 1 cup water

Directions:

1. In a bowl, mix the asparagus with the other ingredients except the water and toss.
2. Put the water in your instant pot, add the steamer basket, put the asparagus sticks inside, put the lid on and cook on High for 6 minutes.
3. Release the pressure fast for 5 minutes, arrange the asparagus on a platter and serve.

Nutrition Values: Calories 181, Fat 6g, Fiber 3g, Carbs 4g, Protein 4g

PORK BITES

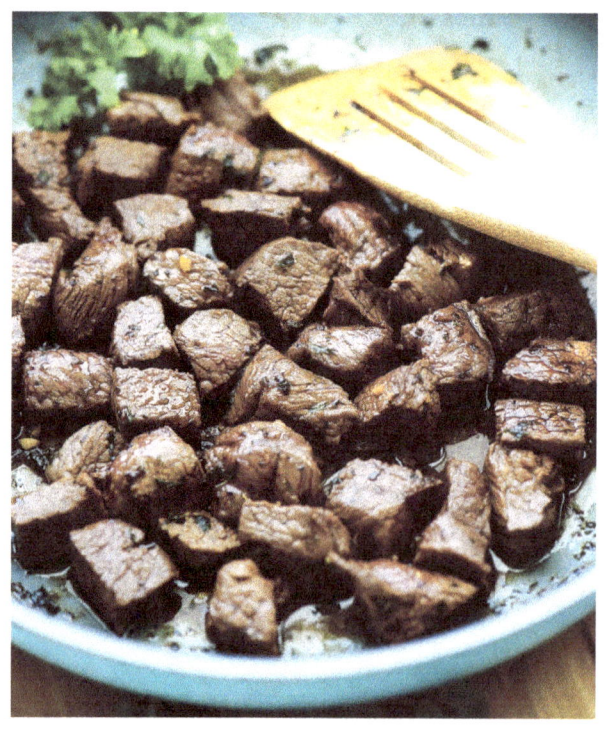

Preparation time: 10 minutes
Cooking time: 30 minutes
Serves: 4

Ingredients:
- 1 pound pork roast, cubed and browned
- 1 tablespoon Italian seasoning
- 1 cup beef stock
- 2 tablespoons water
- 1 tablespoon sweet paprika
- 2 tablespoons tomato sauce
- 1 tablespoon rosemary, chopped

Directions:

1. In your instant pot, combine the pork cubes with the seasoning and the rest of the ingredients except the rosemary, toss, put the lid on and cook on High for 30 minutes.
2. Release the pressure naturally for 10 minutes, arrange the pork cubes on a platter, sprinkle the rosemary on top and serve.

Nutrition Values: Calories 242, Fat 12g, Fiber 2g, Carbs 6g, Protein 14g

Part Five

SALADS & SIDE DISHES

TENDER ROASTED SWEET POTATOES WITH SAVORY TAHINI SAUCE

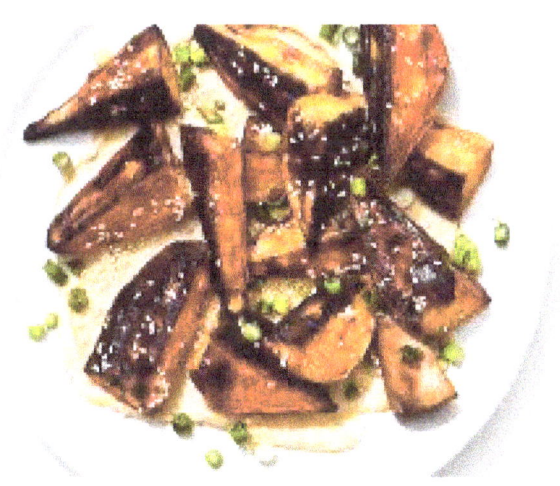

Preparation time: 5 minutes
Cooking time: 30 minutes
Serves: 8

. . .

Ingredients:

- 4 large sweet potatoes, peeled and sliced into half-inch thick coins
- 6 Tbsp. tamarind syrup
- 4 Tbsp. chopped fresh cilantro
- Sea salt
- Extra virgin olive oil
- For the Savory Tahini Sauce:
- 1 1/2 cups tahini
- 1 1/2 Tbsp. freshly squeezed lemon juice
- 1 1/2 Tbsp. Greek yogurt
- 1 1/2 cups water
- 3 garlic cloves, grated
- Sea salt

Directions:

1. First make the tahini sauce by combining all of the ingredients in a bowl and whisking vigorously until creamy. Cover and refrigerate until ready to serve.
2. Set the oven to 450 degrees F. Line a baking sheet with baking paper and set aside.
3. Place the sweet potatoes in a bowl, then drizzle in a bit of olive oil and sprinkle with salt. Spread out on the prepared baking sheet in a single layer, then roast for up to 30 minutes, or until tender and browned.
4. Transfer the roasted sweet potatoes on a serving dish, then spoon the tahini sauce and tamarind syrup on top.
5. Add a drizzle of olive oil, season lightly with salt, garnish with cilantro, then serve right away.

Nutrition Values: Calories 216, Fat 0.4g, Carbohydrates 50.1g, Sugar 40.8g, Protein 0.8g, Cholesterol 0mg

HOMEMADE WHOLE WHEAT PITA BREAD

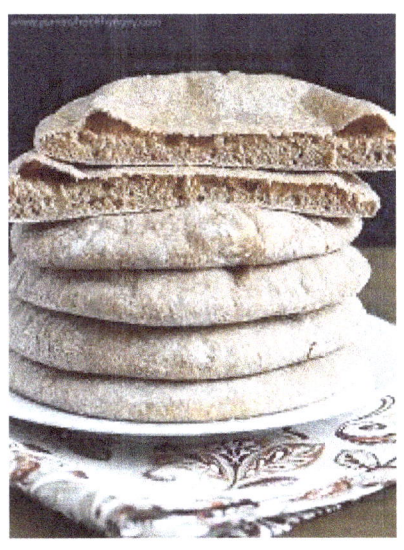

Preparation time: 10 minutes
Cooking time: 2 hours 30 minutes
Serves: 12

. . .

Ingredients:

- 4 cups whole wheat flour (or gluten-free flour)
- 3 cups unbleached all-purpose flour (or gluten-free alternative)
- 2 1/4 cups warm water
- 2 Tbsp. active dry yeast
- 2 Tbsp. extra virgin olive oil
- 1 Tbsp. sea salt

Directions:

1. Combine the yeast and warm water in a very large mixing bowl until thoroughly combined. Stir in the salt.
2. Gradually stir in the two flours into the mixture until you get a dough.
3. Lightly flour a clean, dry surface and place the dough on top. Knead until the dough becomes smooth.
4. Add the olive oil into a large bowl and place the dough on top. Turn the dough several times to coat in the oil. Lightly oil one side of a sheet of plastic wrap, then cover over the bowl. Place a clean kitchen towel over the bowl, then set aside for about 2 hours to rise.
5. Punch down on the risen dough, then divide into 12 pieces. Roll up into balls and arrange on a lightly floured surface. Cover with a clean kitchen towel and allow to rise for about 15 minutes.
6. Set the oven to 475 degrees F. Place a baking sheet on the lowest rack inside.
7. Roll out each ball of dough until each is approximately 6 inches in diameter. Take the baking sheet out of the oven and arrange the unbaked pita on top; do not overcrowd. Bake in batches, if needed.
8. Bake for 12 minutes, then place on a platter. Consume within 3 days.

Nutrition Values: Calories 173, Fat 10.8 g, Carbohydrates 17.8 g, Sugar 2.3 g, Protein 2.2 g, Cholesterol 0 mg

CRISP SPICED CAULIFLOWER WITH FETA CHEESE

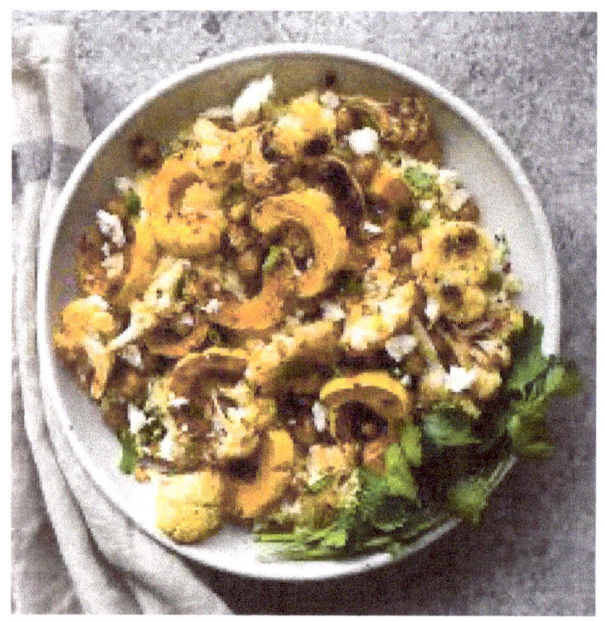

Preparation time: 5 minutes
Cooking time: 10 minutes

Serves: 4

Ingredients:

- 3/4 lb cauliflower, chopped
- 1/2 Tbsp. ground toasted cumin seeds
- 1 garlic clove, grated
- 2 Tbsp. crumbled feta cheese
- 1 1/2 Tbsp. freshly squeezed lemon juice
- 1 Tbsp. chopped fresh flat leaf parsley
- Chili flakes
- Sweet smoked paprika
- Sea salt
- Canola oil

Directions:

1. Place a skillet over high flame and heat just enough canola oil to cover the bottom.
2. Allow the oil to smoke slightly, then add the chopped cauliflower and stir fry for about 2 minutes or until browned and crisp. Season with salt.
3. Reduce to medium flame as you continue to stir fry the cauliflower. Sprinkle in the cumin, lemon juice, grated garlic, and a dash of chili flakes, then stir well to combine.
4. Transfer the cauliflower to a platter, then top with feta, parsley, and a dash of paprika. Serve right away.

Nutrition Values: Calories 300, Fat 19.3 g, Carbohydrates 30.6 g, Sugar 8.8 g, Protein 3.4 g, Cholesterol 0 mg

SPRING PEAS AND BEANS WITH ZESTY THYME YOGURT SAUCE

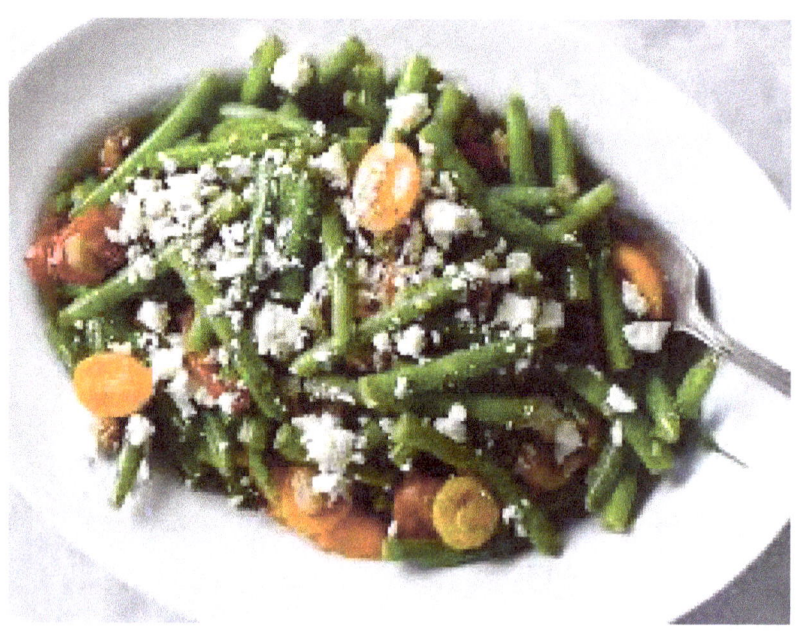

Preparation time: 5 minutes
Cooking time: 10 minutes
Serves: 4

Ingredients:

- 3/4 lb fresh shelling beans, shelled
- 3/4 lb fresh peas (such as English peas, edamame, etc.), shelled
- 1 lb pole beans, preferably assorted (such as purple wax, Romano, and yellow)
- 6 young pea shoots
- 1/2 tsp. ground sumac
- 1 1/2 Tbsp. extra virgin olive oil
- Sea salt
- For the Zesty Thyme Yogurt Sauce:
- 1/4 cup Greek yogurt
- 1 1/2 Tbsp. fresh thyme leaves
- 1 garlic clove, grated
- 1/2 lemon, juiced and zested
- Cayenne
- Sea salt

Directions:

1. Combine all the ingredients for the yogurt sauce in a bowl, then season to taste with salt and cayenne. Cover the bowl and refrigerate until ready to serve.
2. Prepare a bowl of ice water and set aside.
3. Boil some salted water in a saucepan, then add the fresh beans and peas. Boil for 2 minutes, or until tender, then remove immediately with a metal mesh strainer and plunge into the ice water to prevent them from being soggy.
4. Blot the peas and beans dry using paper towels, then place in a large bowl and set aside.

5. Refill the bowl of ice water.
6. Boil the salted water in the saucepan again, then add the pole beans and cook for 2 minutes or until almost tender. Remove immediately with a metal mesh strainer and plunge into the ice water to prevent them from being soggy.
7. Blot the pole beans dry using paper towels, then add to the bowl of peas and beans. Toss everything to combine.
8. Drizzle the olive oil over the peas and beans, then season with salt and sumac. Toss well to combine, then add the yogurt sauce on top. Garnish with pea shoots and thyme, then serve right away.

Nutrition Values: Calories 153, Fat 0.5 g, Carbohydrates 39.1 g, Sugar 25.7 g, Protein 1.2 g, Cholesterol 0 mg

MEDITERRANEAN PASTA SALAD

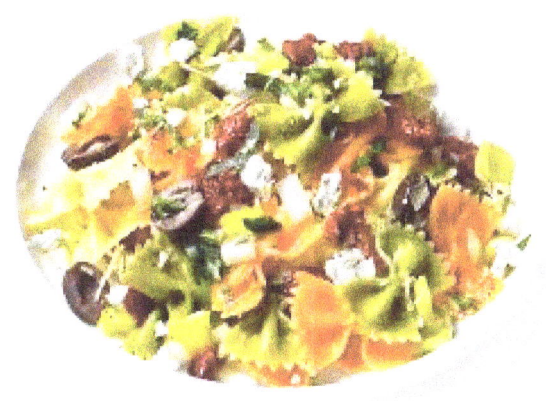

Preparation time: 5 minutes
Cooking time: 30 minutes
Serves: 4

. . .

Ingredients

- Kosher salt
- 1 pound tricolor pasta, such as bow tie or fusilli
- 1/4 cup balsamic vinegar
- 2 to 3 teaspoons dijon mustard
- Freshly ground pepper
- 2/3 to 3/4 cup extra-virgin olive oil
- 1/3 cup diced sun-dried tomatoes
- 1/4 cup fresh basil, julienned
- 1/4 cup diced onion
- 2 large pickled pepperoncini peppers, diced
- 3 tablespoons halved black olives
- 2 teaspoons chopped fresh oregano
- 1 1/2 ounces feta cheese, crumbled
- 1 1/2 tablespoons grated romano cheese

Directions

1. Bring a large pot of salted water to a boil. Add the pasta and cook until al dente; drain, then rinse with cold water to cool.
2. Meanwhile, make the vinaigrette: Whisk the vinegar, mustard, 1 teaspoon salt, and pepper to taste in a small bowl.
3. Gradually whisk in enough of the oil to make a smooth dressing; season with salt and pepper.
4. Combine the sun-dried tomatoes, basil, onion, pepperoncini, olives and oregano in a bowl. Add the cooked pasta, 1/2 teaspoon salt and 1 teaspoon pepper.
5. Add the vinaigrette and both cheeses and toss. Chill until ready to serve.

Nutrition Values: Calories 433, Fat 25.1 g, Carbohydrates 41.4 g, Sugar 10.3 g, Protein 7.8 g, Cholesterol 164 mg

MEDITERRANEAN FARRO SALAD

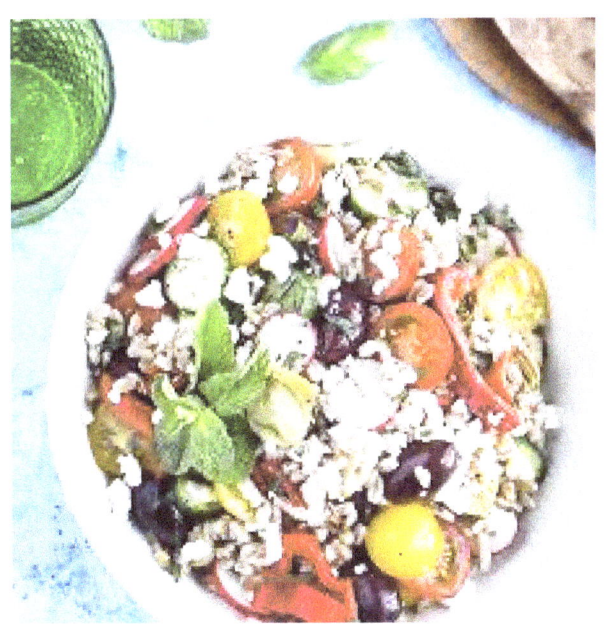

Preparation time: 10 minutes
Cooking time: 34 minutes
Serves: 8

Ingredients

- 10 ounces farro (about 1 1/2 cups)
- 1 1/2 teaspoons kosher salt, plus 1/2 teaspoon
- 8 ounces green beans, cut into 1- to 2-inch pieces (about 2 cups)
- 1/2 cup pitted black olives
- 1 medium red pepper, cut into thin strips (about 4 ounces or 1 cup)
- 3 ounces Parmesan, crumbled (about 3/4 cup)
- 1 small bunch chives, snipped (about 1/4 cup)
- 1/4 cup sherry vinegar
- 1/4 cup extra-virgin olive oil
- 1 tablespoon Dijon mustard
- 1 teaspoon freshly ground black pepper

Directions

1. In a medium saucepan, combine 4 cups of water with the farro. Bring to a boil over high heat. Cover and simmer over medium-low heat until the farro is almost tender, about 20 minutes. Add 1 1/2 teaspoons of the salt and simmer until the farro is tender, about 10 minutes longer. Drain well. Transfer to a large bowl and let cool.
2. Meanwhile, bring a medium pot of salted water to a boil over high heat.
3. Add the green beans and stir. Cook for 2 minutes. Transfer the cooked green beans to a bowl of ice water and let cool for 2 minutes. Drain the green beans.
4. Once the farro has cooled add the green beans, olives, red pepper, Parmesan, and chives. Stir to combine. In a small

bowl mix together the sherry vinegar, olive oil, mustard, pepper, and the remaining 1/2 teaspoon salt.
5. Stir to combine. Pour the sherry vinaigrette over the farro salad. Toss to combine and serve.

Nutrition Values: Calories 452, Fat 24.6 g, Carbohydrates 55.1 g, Sugar 15.3 g, Protein 5.4 g, Cholesterol 0 mg

MEDITERRANEAN COUSCOUS

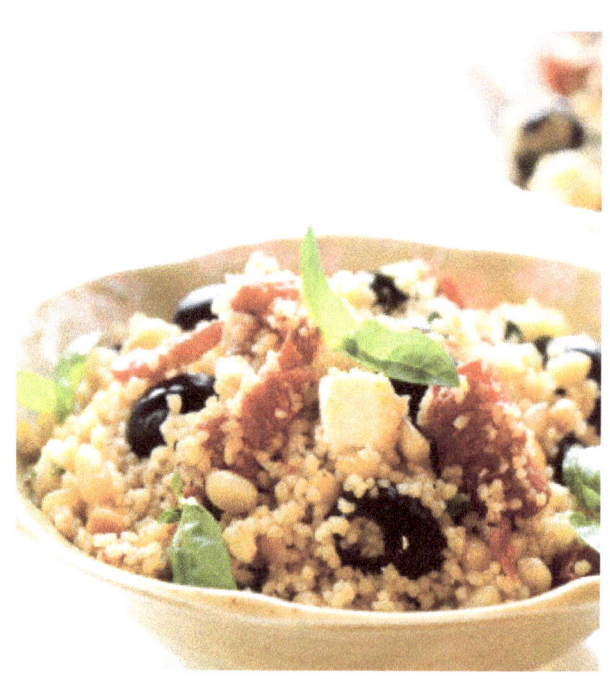

Preparation time: 5 minutes
Cooking time: 10 minutes
Serves: 8

Ingredients

- 1 1/2 cup instant couscous
- 2 cups low-sodium chicken stock
- 4 ounces dried apricots, about 12, finely diced
- Kosher salt and freshly cracked black pepper
- 1/4 cup pitted kalamata olives, chopped
- 3 scallions, thinly sliced

Directions

1. Put the couscous in a large mixing bowl. Put the chicken stock and apricots in a saucepan, season with salt and pepper, and bring to a boil over medium-high heat. Pour the boiling liquid over the couscous, and shake the bowl to moisten every grain.
2. Sprinkle the olives and scallions over the top and cover the bowl tightly with plastic wrap. Let stand 10 minutes, until the liquid is absorbed.
3. To serve, season the couscous with salt and pepper and fluff with a fork. Serve warm or at room temperature.

Nutrition Values: Calories 335, Fat 0.5 g, Carbohydrates 42.1 g, Sugar 25 g, Protein 1.2 g

LOADED MEDITERRANEAN CAULIFLOWER FRIES

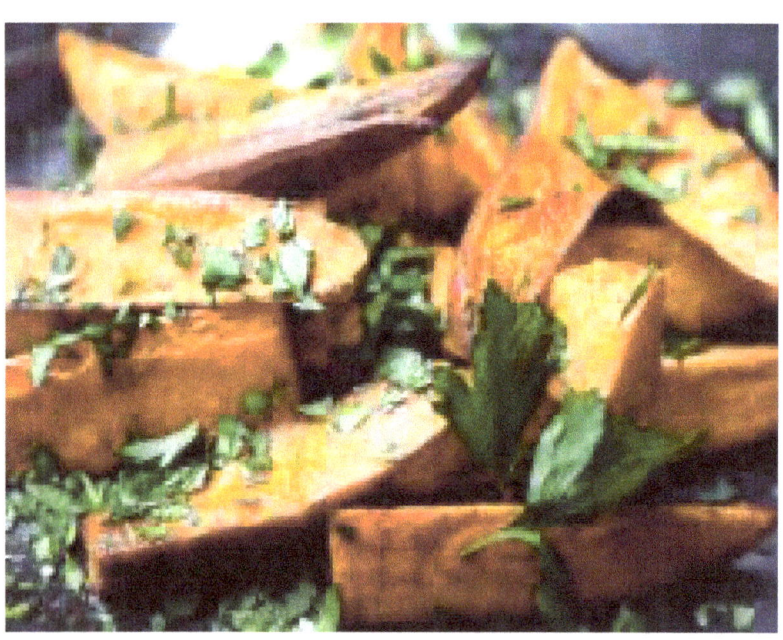

PREPARATION TIME: 5 MINUTES
COOKING TIME: 30 MINUTES
SERVES: 4

Ingredients

- Loaded Fries:
- One 12-ounce bag frozen cauliflower fries
- 1 tablespoon plus 1 1/2 teaspoons za'atar
- Kosher salt and freshly cracked black pepper
- 1/2 cup fresh parsley, leaves torn with your hands
- 1/4 cup finely diced red onion
- 1/4 cup chopped kalamata olives
- 1/4 cup extra-virgin olive oil
- 3 tablespoons chopped pickled pepperoncini
- 1 medium cucumber, finely diced
- 1/3 cup crumbled feta
- Yogurt Sauce:
- 1 cup plain whole-milk Greek yogurt
- 1/2 cup fresh mint, chopped
- 3 tablespoons chopped capers
- 1/2 teaspoon ground coriander
- Zest of 1 lemon plus juice of up to 2 lemons
- Hot sauce, to taste
- Kosher salt and freshly cracked black pepper

Directions

1. For the loaded fries: Preheat the oven to 425 degrees F. Put a baking sheet in the oven for 10 minutes to heat up.
2. Toss the frozen cauliflower fries with 1 tablespoon of the za'atar and season with salt and pepper. Place on the hot baking sheet and bake until crispy and hot, 13 to 15 minutes depending on your oven.
3. While the fries are cooking, in a medium bowl, combine the

parsley, onion, olives, olive oil, pepperoncini, cucumber and the remaining 1 1/2 teaspoons za'atar. Season with pepper (the olives are salty).
4. For the yogurt sauce: Combine the yogurt, mint, capers, coriander, lemon zest and juice and some hot sauce in a small mixing bowl. You may add more or less lemon juice depending on how thick your yogurt is, or how tart you would like your sauce. Season with salt and pepper.
5. To finish, spread the yogurt sauce on the bottom of a plate. Place the crispy fries on top of the sauce. Top with the cucumber-olive salad and finish with the crumbled feta.

Nutrition Values: Calories 115, Fat 8g, Carbohydrates 115g, Protein 4g

MEDITERRANEAN SUCCOTASH

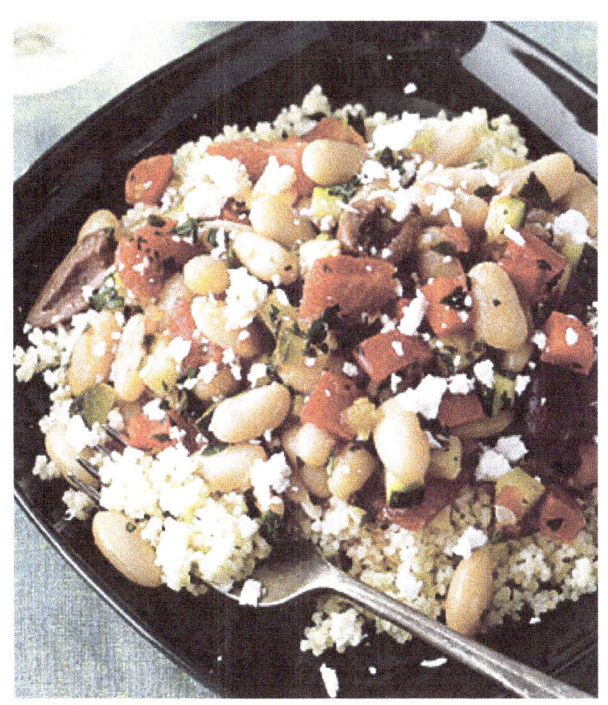

Preparation time: 5 minutes
Cooking time: 12 minutes
Serves: 5

Ingredients

- 2 tablespoons extra-virgin olive oil, 2 turns of the pan
- 1 red onion, diced
- 2 cloves garlic, chopped
- 2 bell peppers, yellow, red, and/or green, seeded and chopped
- 1 bunch asparagus, sliced on bias, tips 1 1/2 inches long
- 2 cups frozen corn kernels
- 1 can butter beans, drained
- Salt and pepper
- Handful flat-leaf parsley, chopped

Directions

1. Heat a medium skillet over medium high heat. Add oil, onion, garlic, peppers.
2. Saute peppers, stirring frequently, 5 minutes. Add asparagus and corn, cook 3 to 5 minutes longer. Add beans and heat them through, 1 or 2 minutes.
3. Season dish with salt and pepper, to your taste, then stir in parsley. Transfer to dinner plates or bowls and serve.

Nutrition Values: Calories 115, Fat 8g, Carbohydrates 115g, Protein 4g

MEDITERRANEAN COUSCOUS SALAD

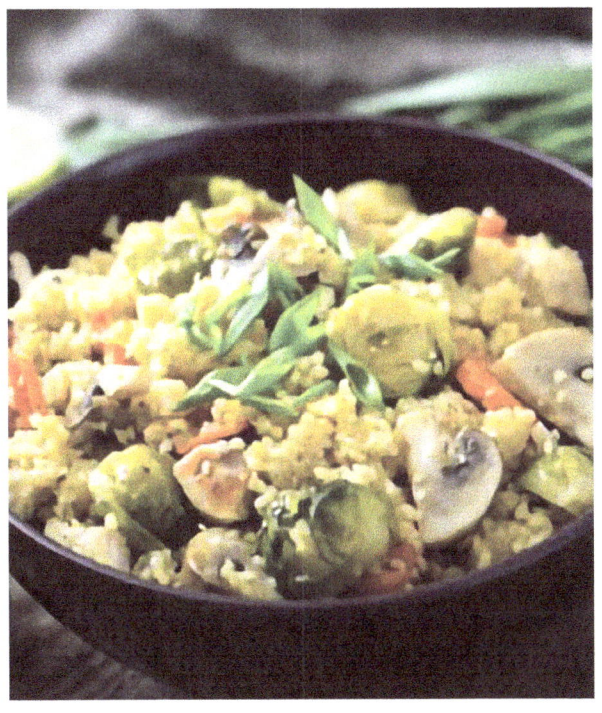

Preparation time: 5 minutes
Cooking time: 30 minutes
Serves: 3

Ingredients

- 2 tablespoons olive oil (1 tablespoon for the tomatoes and 1 tablespoon to toss with the couscous)
- 4 yellow tomatoes
- 1 pound Israeli couscous (pearl pasta)
- 1 red bell pepper, stems and seeds removed and cut brunoise
- 1/2 cup fresh mint leaves, packed plus a few small sprigs for garnish
- 1 (8-ounce) jar pickled cipollini onions
- 2 English cucumbers, peeled and sliced into 1/4-inch thick disks

Dressing:

- 2 tablespoons red wine vinegar
- 2 garlic cloves, lightly crushed with the side of a knife blade and quartered
- 1 teaspoon Dijon mustard
- 1/2 teaspoon salt
- 1/2 teaspoon black pepper
- 1/2 cup extra-virgin olive oil

Directions

1. Preheat oven to 325 degrees F. Brush 1 tablespoon olive oil on the tomatoes (reserving the rest) and roast for about 25 minutes. Remove from oven, allow cooling, and cut into wedges.
2. Boil couscous until al dente as you would for pasta, drain well, and toss with 1 tablespoon reserved olive oil.

3. For the dressing, add the vinegar to a blender and replace the cover. Turn on the blender and through the feed opening add, 1 at a time, the garlic, mustard, salt, and pepper. Leaving the blender running, add the olive oil in a slow thin stream. Set aside briefly.
4. Toss together the couscous, tomatoes, bell pepper, mint leaves, cipollini onions, and cucumber with enough of the dressing to coat. Serve additional dressing on the side.

Nutrition Values: Calories 270, Fat 22g, Carbohydrates 11g, Protein 9g

MEDITERRANEAN BARLEY SALAD

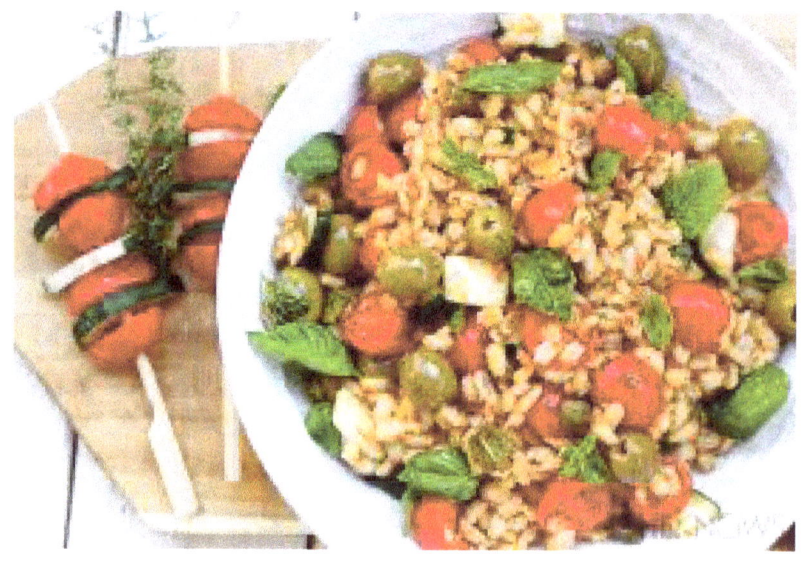

Preparation time: 10 minutes
Cooking time: 40 minutes
Serves: 4

. . .

Ingredients

Salad:

- 2 cups vegetable broth, low-sodium canned, or homemade
- 1 cup barley
- 1 teaspoon extra-virgin olive oil
- 1 teaspoon kosher salt
- 1/2 cup chopped Kalamata olives
- 2 medium tomatoes, diced
- 1/2 English cucumber, diced
- 2/3 cup chopped flat-leaf parsley

Dressing:

- 1/2 cup fresh lemon juice
- 1/4 teaspoon kosher salt
- Freshly ground black pepper
- 3 tablespoons extra-virgin olive oil

Directions

1. Bring broth to a boil in a medium saucepan. Add the barley, oil, and salt. Bring back to a boil, adjust heat to maintain a gentle simmer, cover and cook until tender, about 30 minutes.
2. Remove from the heat and let stand, covered, for 10 minutes more. Drain excess liquid, if needed. Cool.
3. Meanwhile, whisk the lemon juice, salt, and pepper in a large serving bowl.
4. Gradually whisk in the oil, starting with a few drops and then adding the rest in a steady stream, to make a smooth dressing.
5. Add the barley and the remaining salad ingredients and toss to coat with the dressing. Serve.

Nutrition Values: Calories 57, Fat 5g, Carbohydrates 2g, Protein 2g

TABBOULEH

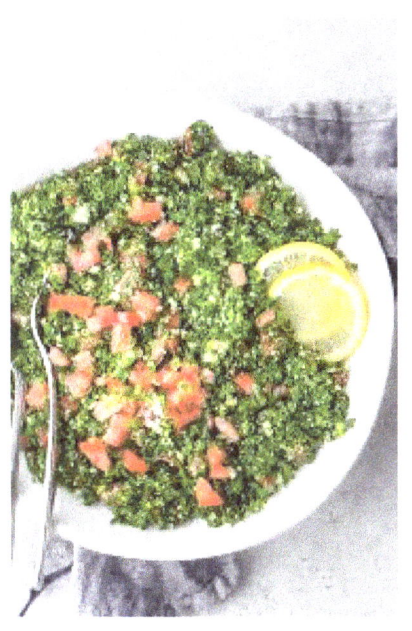

Preparation time: 10 minutes
Cooking time: 60 minutes

Serves: 4

Ingredients

- 1 cup bulgur wheat
- 1 1/2 cups boiling water
- 1/4 cup freshly squeezed lemon juice (2 lemons)
- 1/4 cup good olive oil
- 3 1/2 teaspoons kosher salt
- 1 cup minced scallions, white and green parts (1 bunch)
- 1 cup chopped fresh mint leaves (1 bunch)
- 1 cup chopped flat-leaf parsley (1 bunch)
- 1 hothouse cucumber, unpeeled, seeded, and medium-diced
- 2 cups cherry tomatoes, cut in half
- 1 teaspoon freshly ground black pepper

Directions

1. Place the bulgur in a large bowl, pour in the boiling water, and add the lemon juice, olive oil, and 1 1/2 teaspoons salt. Stir, then allow to stand at room temperature for about 1 hour.
2. Add the scallions, mint, parsley, cucumber, tomatoes, 2 teaspoons salt, and the pepper; mix well. Season, to taste, and serve or cover and refrigerate. The flavor will improve if the tabbouleh sits for a few hours.

Nutrition Values: Calories 371, Fat 18g, Carbohydrates 43g, Protein 8g

SPINACH SALAD WITH GRILLED MEDITERRANEAN VEGETABLES

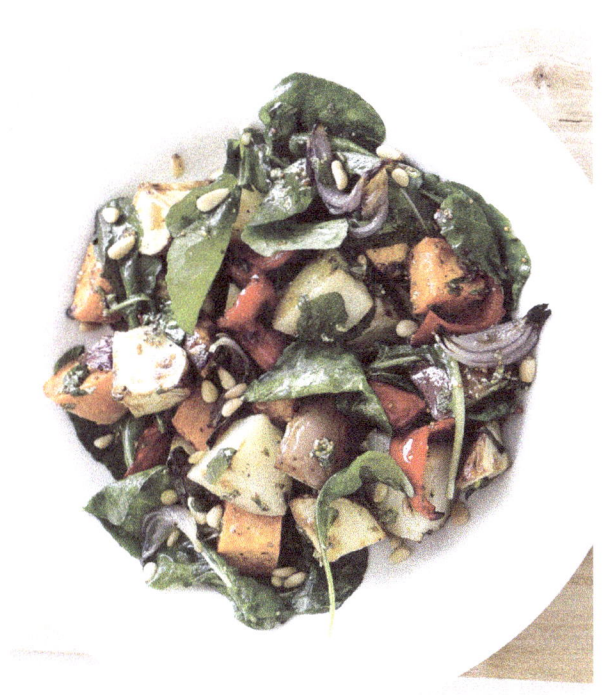

Preparation time: 5 minutes
Cooking time: 10 minutes
Serves: 4

Ingredients

- 1 small orange bell pepper, seeded and quartered
- 2 large Portobello mushroom caps, stemmed, sliced
- 1 small summer squash, cut on bias
- 1 (14-ounce) can artichoke hearts, drained, rinsed and quartered
- 1/4 cup olive oil, plus more to taste
- Salt and freshly ground black pepper
- 1/2 cup feta cheese, diced
- 1/4 cup kalamata olives, pitted
- 3 cups baby spinach
- 1 cup packed basil leaves

Directions

1. Place all vegetables in a large mixing bowl. Add 1/4 cup oil and season with salt and pepper, to taste. Toss well making sure each vegetable gets covered with oil. Place a grill pan over medium heat. Once heated, place your vegetables on grill and cook accordingly: grill mushrooms about 5 minutes per side; peppers and squash about 3 minutes per side.
2. Once all the vegetables are grilled place them in a large serving bowl to slightly cool. Dice and add feta cheese, pitted olives, spinach and basil leaves. Gently toss to mix well and drizzle more oil, to taste, if necessary and serve.

Nutrition Values: Calories 200, Fat 6g, Fiber 2g, Carbs 5g, Protein 6g

MEDITERRANEAN CHICKEN SAMOSAS WITH APPLE CUMIN CHUTNEY

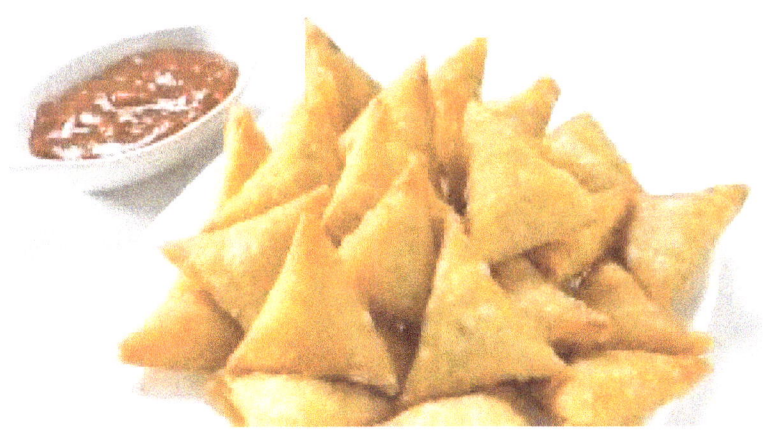

Preparation time: 10 minutes
Cooking time: 33 minutes
Serves: 3

Ingredients

- Apple Cumin Chutney:
- 1/2 white onion, diced
- 1 green apple, peeled and cored
- 1 tablespoon gari, chopped
- 1 tablespoon brown sugar
- 1 teaspoon ground cumin
- Salt and pepper
- Plain yogurt

Samosas:

- Vegetable oil
- 1 pound chicken thighs, ground
- 3/4 cup finely diced white onion (about 1/2 onion)
- 3/4 tablespoon garlic puree (about 2 cloves)
- 1 tablespoon ground cumin
- 1/2 teaspoon chili flakes
- 1 cup grated Asiago cheese
- 1/4 bunch fresh sage leaves, julienned
- 16 to 20 spring roll wrappers
- 1 egg, beaten

Directions

1. For the chutney: In a saucepan over medium heat, sweat the onions until softened, about 4 minutes. Add the green apples and reduce the heat to low and cook until the apples soften, about 5 minutes. Add the gari, sugar, cumin, and salt and pepper to taste. Once completely softened, it only takes a couple minutes, puree everything in a food processor. Let cool. Once the mixture is cooled, add equal parts yogurt and puree again. The chutney can be refrigerated for up to 4 days.
2. For the samosas: In a preheated saucepan over medium-high

heat, add a little bit of vegetable oil and brown the chicken with the onions, garlic puree, cumin and chili flakes, about 15 minutes. The chicken will render liquid as will the onions. Once browned and fully cooked through, season with salt and pepper. Let cool. Then, add the Asiago and sage. Set aside. Cut the spring roll wrappers in half, creating two long, rectangle-shaped strips.
3. Using a pastry brush, place egg wash on the top half of the strip. Add about 1 tablespoon of the chicken filling to the bottom half of the strip (the half that does not have the egg wash).
4. Starting at the bottom, fold the wrapper at a 45-degree angle, making triangles over and over as you work your way up, similar to folding spanakopita. Apply egg wash if needed to seal the edges once you are done folding the wrapper.
5. Heat a deep pot with oil to 350 degrees F. Deep-fry the samosas until lightly browned and crispy, 3 to 4 minutes.
6. Then drain on paper towels and season with salt and pepper while the samosas are still hot and wet. Serve the apple cumin chutney on the side with the samosas.

Nutrition Values: Calories 200, Fat 5g, Fiber 2g, Carbs 5g, Protein 6g

TOASTED ISRAELI COUSCOUS WITH VEGETABLES AND LEMON-BALSAMIC VINAIGRETTE

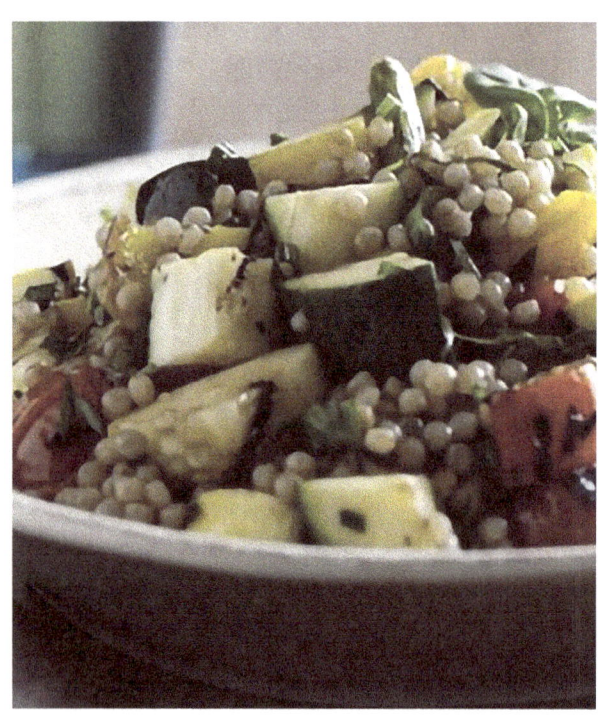

Preparation time: 5 minutes
Cooking time: 40 minutes
Serves: 4

Ingredients

- 1/2 pound Israeli couscous
- Salt
- 12 spears asparagus, grilled and cut into 1/4-inch pieces
- 1 zucchini, halved, grilled and cut into 1-inch pieces
- 1 yellow squash, halved, grilled and cut into 1-inch pieces
- 2 large red peppers, grilled, peeled and diced into bite-size pieces
- 1/2 cup kalamata olives, pitted and chopped
- 2 tablespoons chopped fresh basil leaves
- Freshly ground black pepper
- Lemon-Balsamic Vinaigrette, recipe follows
- Lemon-Balsamic Vinaigrette:
- 1 small shallot, minced
- 3 tablespoons fresh lemon juice
- 1 teaspoon lemon zest
- 3 tablespoons aged balsamic vinegar
- 1 tablespoon red wine vinegar
- Salt and freshly ground black pepper
- 3/4 cup extra-virgin olive oil

Directions

1. Heat large saute pan on grates of the grill over medium heat. Add couscous and toast until lightly golden brown.
2. Bring 6 cups of water to a boil over high heat, add 1 tablespoon salt and toasted couscous and cook until al dente. Drain well and place in a large bowl. Add grilled vegetables, olives, basil, and vinaigrette and toss until combined; season with salt and pepper. Let sit at room

temperature for 30 minutes before serving or cover and refrigerate.
3. Lemon-Balsamic Vinaigrette:
4. Whisk shallot, juice, zest, vinegars, and salt and pepper together in a small bowl. Slowly whisk in oil until emulsified.

Nutrition Values: Calories 200, Fat 4g, Fiber 2g, Carbs 6g, Protein 6g

ELBOW MACARONI WITH PINE NUTS, LEMON AND FENNEL

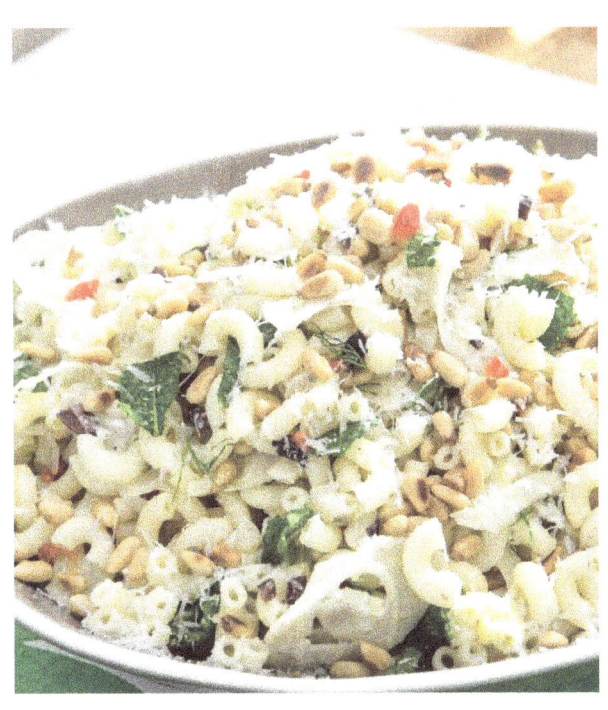

Preparation time: 5 minutes
Cooking time: 30 minutes
Serves: 2

Ingredients

- Kosher salt
- 1/4 cup red wine vinegar
- 1/2 cup plus 2 tablespoons extra-virgin olive oil
- 1/2 cup toasted Mediterranean pine nuts
- 2 tablespoons finely chopped kalamata olives
- 1 tablespoon minced red cherry peppers
- 1 tablespoon chopped capers
- Finely grated zest and juice of 1 lemon (about 3 tablespoons juice)
- 1 small fennel bulb, trimmed, cored and thinly sliced, plus 1/2 cup fennel fronds, coarsely chopped
- 1/4 cup chopped fresh mint leaves
- 3 cups elbow macaroni (about 12 ounces)
- 1/2 cup freshly grated Pecorino-Romano

Directions

1. Bring a large pot of salted water to a boil.
2. In a large bowl, add the vinegar and 1/2 cup of the oil. Add the pine nuts, olives, cherry pepper, capers and lemon zest. Toss the sliced fennel with the lemon juice and a pinch of salt in a small bowl. Combine the fennel with the dressing mixture. Add the fennel fronds and mint. Season with pepper. Let it sit while you cook the pasta.
3. Add the pasta to the boiling water and cook according to package directions until al dente. Drain, rinse and pat dry on a sheet pan lined with a kitchen towel. In a large bowl, toss with the remaining 2 tablespoons oil.

4. Add the pasta to the fennel mixture and stir to combine. Season with salt and pepper. Sprinkle the pasta with the cheese. Serve room temperature.

Nutrition Values: Calories 162, Fat 3g, Fiber 2g, Carbs 5g, Protein 6g

VEGETABLE COUSCOUS

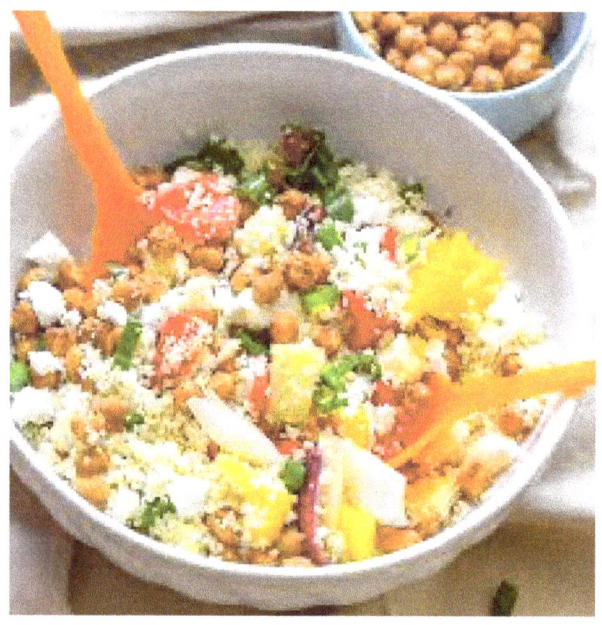

Preparation time: 5 minutes
Cooking time: 13 minutes

SERVES: 4

Ingredients

- 2 tablespoon extra-virgin olive oil
- 1 bay leaf, fresh or dried
- 1 medium onion, chopped
- 1/4 zucchini, diced
- 1/4 yellow squash, diced
- Salt and pepper
- 1/2 cup canned pumpkin
- 4 cups chicken or vegetable broth
- 1 1/2 teaspoons ground cumin, half a palm full
- 1 teaspoon coriander seeds, 1 /3 palm full
- 2 1/4 cups couscous
- 1 vine ripe plum tomato, seeded and finely chopped
- 2 tablespoons each chopped cilantro and flat-leaf parsley
- Mediterranean flatbread, for passing

Directions

1. Heat a large sauce pot over medium high heat. Add oil, bay leaf, onion, zucchini and yellow squash to the pot and season with salt and pepper.
2. Saute, stirring frequently, 7 or 8 minutes. Add pumpkin and broth to the pan and stir to combine. Add cumin and coriander. Bring broth to a boil.
3. Add couscous to the broth, stir, cover and remove from heat. Let stand 5 minutes. Remove lid from the pot and fluff couscous with a fork.
4. Remove bay from the pan, add finely chopped tomato, cilantro and parsley, toss again with fork to combine and transfer to a serving platter.
5. Serve with warm Mediterranean flatbreads.

Nutrition Values: Calories 128, Fat 5g, Fiber 1g, Carbs 2g, Protein 6g

SAFFRON RICE SALAD

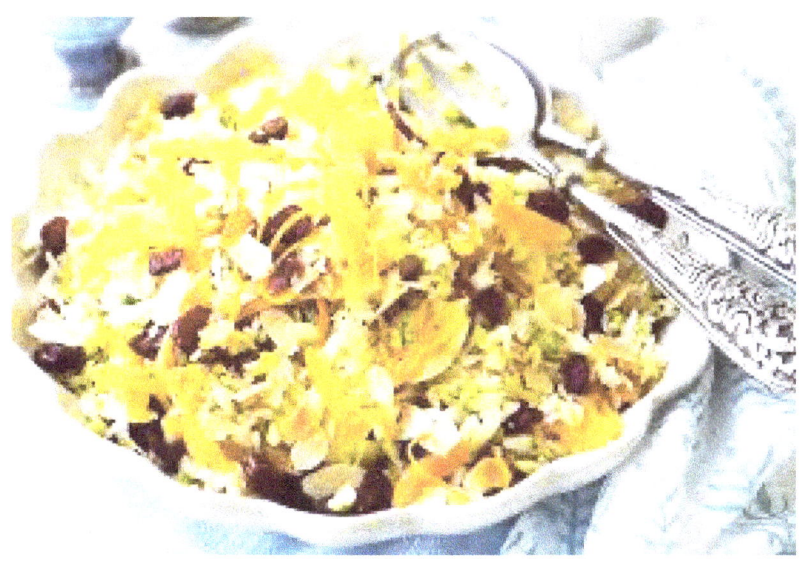

Preparation time: 5 minutes
Cooking time: 20 minutes
Serves: 3

. . .

Ingredients

- 3 tablespoons olive oil, plus more for dressing
- 1 Spanish onion, finely chopped
- 2 cloves garlic, finely chopped
- 2 cups long grain white rice
- 4 cups water
- 1 large pinch saffron threads
- Salt and freshly ground pepper
- 8 spears asparagus, grilled and cut into 1/2-inch pieces
- 1 red pepper, fire roasted and diced
- 1 yellow pepper, fire roasted and diced
- 3/4 cup salt cured olives, pitted and chopped
- 1/4 cup chopped fresh herbs, ie: parsley or cilantro leaves
- Extra-virgin olive oil, for drizzling
- 2 tablespoons aged Sherry vinegar

Directions

1. Heat oil in medium pot on grates of grill or side burners. Add onions and garlic and cook until soft. Add the rice and stir to coat the grains of rice with the oil.
2. Place the water in a small pot and bring to a boil. Add the saffron to the onion mixture and let boil 1 minute. Add the boiling water to the rice, stir, add salt and pepper and bring to a boil. Reduce the heat to medium-low, cover the pot and let cook 12 to 14 minutes or until the rice is just cooked. Let the rice sit covered for 5 minutes then fluff with fork.
3. Transfer the rice to a large bowl and add the asparagus, peppers, olives and herbs. Drizzle with extra-virgin olive oil and a few tablespoons of aged sherry vinegar. Serve warm or at room temperature.

Nutrition Values: Calories 187, Fat 4g, Fiber 2g, Carbs 4g, Protein 6g

LEMON RICE

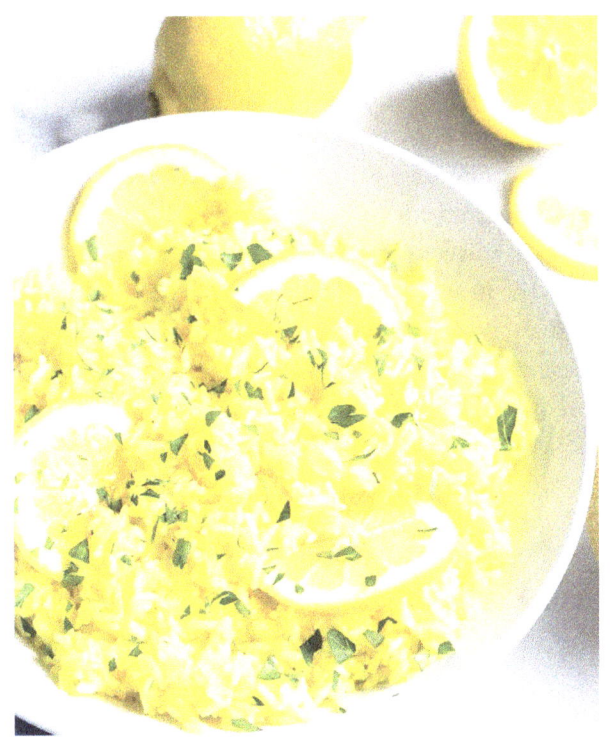

Preparation time: 5 minutes
Cooking time: 25 minutes
Serves: 8

Ingredients

- 1 tablespoon vegetable oil
- 1 small yellow onion, finely diced
- 2 cups long-grain white rice
- Kosher salt
- 1/4 cup fresh lemon juice
- 3 tablespoons chopped fresh mint, plus more for garnish

Directions

1. Heat the oil in a medium saucepan over medium heat. Add the onions and cook until soft, taking care not to let them color, 3 to 5 minutes.
2. Add the rice and stir to coat with the oil.
3. Add 3 cups water and 1 teaspoon salt and bring to a boil. Reduce the heat to low, then cover and cook until all of the liquid has been absorbed, about 20 minutes. Remove from the heat and fluff with a fork to separate the grains. Let sit, covered, for 5 to 10 minutes.
4. Add the lemon juice and mint to the rice and toss to distribute evenly.
5. Serve hot, garnished with chopped mint.

Nutrition Values: Calories 200, Fat 7g, Fiber 2g, Carbs 4g, Protein 6g

CARROT SLAW

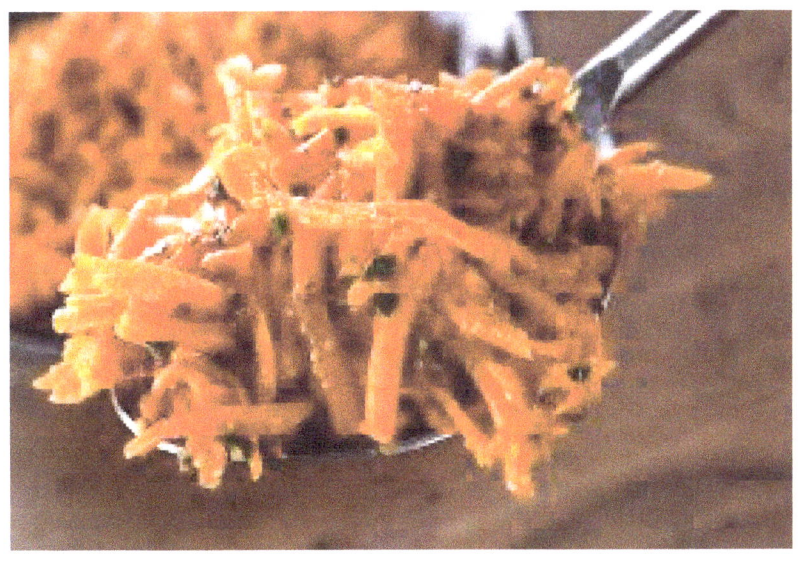

Preparation time: 35 minutes
Cooking time: 0 minutes
Serves: 8

. . .

Ingredients

- 2 tablespoons freshly squeezed lemon juice
- 2 tablespoons white wine vinegar
- 1 teaspoon Dijon mustard
- Pinch crushed red pepper flakes
- Kosher salt and freshly ground black pepper
- Kosher salt and freshly ground black pepper
- 3 tablespoons olive oil
- 3 large carrots, peeled and shredded
- 2 tablespoons chopped fresh parsley

Directions

1. In a small bowl, whisk together the lemon juice, vinegar, mustard, red pepper flakes and some salt and pepper until smooth.
2. Whisk in the olive oil until completely blended.
3. Toss the shredded carrots with the dressing in a large bowl. Taste and season with more salt or pepper as needed. Add the parsley and toss.
4. Chill 30 minutes before serving.

Nutrition Values: Calories 142, Fat 2g, Fiber 2g, Carbs 4g, Protein 6g

GREEK SALAD WITH SAGANAKI

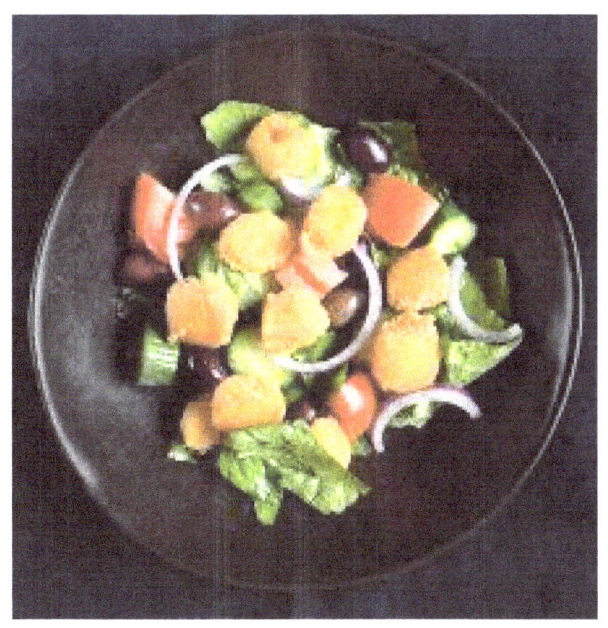

Preparation time: 5 minutes
Cooking time: 30 minutes
Serves: 8

Ingredients

- 3 heads Romaine lettuce, washed and torn into bite sized pieces
- 1 pint grape tomatoes, halved
- 1 cup kalamata olives
- 1 cucumber, sliced
- Greek vinaigrette, recipe follows
- 12 pepperoncini
- 2 small red onions, thinly sliced

Greek Vinaigrette:

- 1 shallot, diced
- 1/2 cup fresh lemon juice
- 1/4 cup feta cheese, crumbled
- 1/2 teaspoon dried oregano
- 1 teaspoon salt
- Freshly ground pepper
- 1 1/2 cups extra-virgin olive oil

Saganaki:

- 1 pound kasseri cheese, cut into 1/2-inch pieces
- 3 tablespoons butter, melted
- 2 tablespoons brandy
- 1 lemon, juiced

Directions (*Greek Vinaigrette & Saganaki*)

Greek Vinaigrette:

1. Put the shallot into the bowl of a food processor and pulse until well chopped.
2. Add the lemon juice, feta, oregano, salt and pepper and pulse again to combine.
3. With the processor running, add the oil in a steady stream.
4. Pour into a small pitcher and set aside.

Saganaki:

1. Preheat the broiler.
2. Put the kasseri slices onto a baking sheet and brush with the melted butter.
3. Place under the broiler until the cheese starts to bubble, about 4 to 5 minutes.
4. Remove from the oven, douse with the brandy and ignite.
5. Let the flame die down, sprinkle with lemon juice, transfer to a serving platter and serve immediately.

Directions

1. Put all the romaine into a large mixing bowl.
2. Add half of the tomatoes, kalamatas and cucumbers and toss to combine.
3. Put the salad into a large decorative bowl, toss with 1 cup of the vinaigrette and garnish with the remaining tomatoes, cucumbers, pepperoncini, kalamatas, and red onion.
4. Serve with the remaining vinaigrette and Saganaki on the side.

Nutrition Values: Calories 182, Fat 4g, Fiber 2g, Carbs 7g, Protein 5g

21-DAY MEAL PLAN

WEEK 1

Day 1
Breakfast- Breakfast Enchiladas
Lunch- Beef Steaks with Spicy Sauce
Dinner- Baked Salmon in Garlic Pepper

Day 2
Breakfast- Mediterranean Breakfast Wraps
Lunch- Delicious Sausage Kebabs
Dinner- Sauteed Octopus

Day 3
Breakfast- Hearty Breakfast Frittata w/ Tomato Salad
Lunch- Salmon and Creamy Endives
Dinner- Steamed Mussels in Tomato Garlic

Day 4
Breakfast- Spaghetti Frittata
Lunch- Baked Trout and Fennel

Dinner- Mediterranean-style Mussels

Day 5
Breakfast- Hearty Breakfast Frittata w/ Tomato Salad
Lunch- Salmon and Creamy Endives
Dinner- Steamed Mussels in Tomato Garlic

Day 6
Breakfast- Mediterranean Breakfast Wraps
Lunch- Delicious Sausage Kebabs
Dinner- Sauteed Octopus

Day 7
Breakfast- Breakfast Quesadilla
Lunch- Smoked Salmon and Veggies Mix
Dinner- Garlic Shrimp with Olive Oil

SHOPPING LIST FOR WEEK 1

The following list contains a number of food products, from staple items and canned goods, to meats and dairy products, all of which can be found in your local grocery store. Feel free to consult this list the next time you go grocery shopping.

Staple items

- Olive oil
- Extra-virgin olive oil
- Balsamic vinegar
- Parsley Oregano
- Cinnamon
- Basil
- Cumin
- Pepper
- Cloves
- Coriander

- Fennel seeds
- Dill
- Rosemary
- Ginger
- Garlic
- Tahini
- Hummus

Canned and packaged

- Olive
- Whole grain bread
- Canned tomatoes
- Whole grain pasta
- Legumes
- White beans
- Chickpeas
- Black beans
- Red kidney beans
- Buckwheat
- Brown rice
- Whole-wheat couscous
- Barley
- Quinoa
- Faro
- Oats
- Almonds
- Hazelnuts
- Sesame seeds
- Cashews
- Walnuts
- Peanuts
- Pistachios
- Sunflower seeds

Produce

- Eggplants
- Onions
- Tomatoes
- Zucchinis
- Apples
- Mushrooms
- Oranges
- Berries
- Pears
- Grapes
- Bananas
- Artichokes
- Avocado
- Asparagus
- Broccoli
- Dates
- Beets
- Brussels sprouts
- Carrots
- Cabbage
- Cucumbers
- Cherries
- Figs
- Limes
- Mushrooms
- Melons
- Squash
- Spinach
- Pomegranate

Fish and meat

- Chicken
- Tuna
- Salmon
- Haddock

- Mackerel
- Turkey
- Mussels
- Shellfish
- Scallops
- Tilapia
- Clams
- Crab

Dairy and eggs

- Greek yogurt
- Low-fat milk
- Eggs
- Goat cheese
- Parmesan
- Mozzarella

WEEK 2

Day 8
Breakfast- Panera Mediterranean Breakfast Sandwich
Lunch- Turkey Cutlets
Dinner- Grilled Octopus

Day 9
Breakfast- Greek Scramble
Lunch- Slow Cooked Chicken
Dinner- Scallop Salad

Day 10
Breakfast- Cheesy Mediterranean Scramble
Lunch- Mediterranean Meatloaf
Dinner- Delicious Chicken Soup

Day 11

Breakfast- Mediterranean Omelet
Lunch- Chili Calamari and Veggie Mix
Dinner- Classic Mediterranean Chicken Soup

Day 12

Breakfast- Huevos Revueltos
Lunch- Greek Trout Spread
Dinner- Easy Chicken Stew

Day 13

Breakfast- Creamy Cuban Fu Fu
Lunch- Cayenne Cod and Tomatoes
Dinner- Chicken and Cabbage Mix

Day 14

Breakfast- Roasted Asparagus Prosciutto & Egg
Lunch- Shrimp and Dill Mix
Dinner- Mediterranean Chicken and Rice Soup

SHOPPING LIST FOR WEEK 2

The following list contains a number of food products, from staple items and canned goods, to meats and dairy products, all of which can be found in your local grocery store. Feel free to consult this list the next time you go grocery shopping.

Staple items

- Olive oil
- Extra-virgin olive oil
- Balsamic vinegar
- Parsley Oregano
- Cinnamon
- Basil
- Cumin
- Pepper
- Cloves

- Coriander
- Fennel seeds
- Dill
- Rosemary
- Ginger
- Garlic
- Tahini
- Hummus

Canned and packaged

- Olive
- Whole grain bread
- Canned tomatoes
- Whole grain pasta
- Legumes
- White beans
- Chickpeas
- Black beans
- Red kidney beans
- Buckwheat
- Brown rice
- Whole-wheat couscous
- Barley
- Quinoa
- Faro
- Oats
- Almonds
- Hazelnuts
- Sesame seeds
- Cashews
- Walnuts
- Peanuts
- Pistachios
- Sunflower seeds

Produce

- Eggplants
- Onions
- Tomatoes
- Zucchinis
- Apples
- Mushrooms
- Oranges
- Berries
- Pears
- Grapes
- Bananas
- Artichokes
- Avocado
- Asparagus
- Broccoli
- Dates
- Beets
- Brussels sprouts
- Carrots
- Cabbage
- Cucumbers
- Cherries
- Figs
- Limes
- Mushrooms
- Melons
- Squash
- Spinach
- Pomegranate

Fish and meat

- Chicken
- Tuna

- Salmon
- Haddock
- Mackerel
- Turkey
- Mussels
- Shellfish
- Scallops
- Tilapia
- Clams
- Crab

Dairy and eggs

- Greek yogurt
- Low-fat milk
- Eggs
- Goat cheese
- Parmesan
- Mozzarella

WEEK 3

Day 15
Breakfast- Creamy Loaded Mashed Potatoes
Lunch- Salmon & Asparagus
Dinner- Healthy Mediterranean Chicken

Day 16
Breakfast- Mediterranean Tofu Scramble
Lunch- High-Quality Belizean Chicken Stew
Dinner- Mushroom and Chicken Bowl

Day 17
Breakfast- Potato and Zucchini Omelet
Lunch- The Great Poblano Chicken Curry
Dinner- Chicken And Broccoli Platter

Day 18
Breakfast- Secret Breakfast Sundaes
Lunch- The Original Mexican Chicken Cacciatore
Dinner- Daring Salted Baked Chicken

Day 19
Breakfast- Banana Nut Oatmeal
Lunch- Magnificent Chicken Curry Soup
Dinner- Worthy Ghee-Licious Chicken

Day 20
Breakfast- Greek Frittata w/ Zucchini, Tomatoes, Feta, and Herbs
Lunch- Awesome Ligurian Chicken
Dinner- Chicken Korma

Day 21
Breakfast- Greek Yogurt Pancakes
Lunch- Garlic And Lemon Chicken Dish
Dinner- Turkey With Garlic Sauce

SHOPPING LIST FOR WEEK 3

The following list contains a number of food products, from staple items and canned goods, to meats and dairy products, all of which can be found in your local grocery store. Feel free to consult this list the next time you go grocery shopping.

Staple items

- Olive oil
- Extra-virgin olive oil
- Balsamic vinegar
- Parsley Oregano
- Cinnamon
- Basil
- Cumin
- Pepper

- Cloves
- Coriander
- Fennel seeds
- Dill
- Rosemary
- Ginger
- Garlic
- Tahini
- Hummus

Canned and packaged

- Olive
- Whole grain bread
- Canned tomatoes
- Whole grain pasta
- Legumes
- White beans
- Chickpeas
- Black beans
- Red kidney beans
- Buckwheat
- Brown rice
- Whole-wheat couscous
- Barley
- Quinoa
- Faro
- Oats
- Almonds
- Hazelnuts
- Sesame seeds
- Cashews
- Walnuts
- Peanuts
- Pistachios
- Sunflower seeds

Produce

- Eggplants
- Onions
- Tomatoes
- Zucchinis
- Apples
- Mushrooms
- Oranges
- Berries
- Pears
- Grapes
- Bananas
- Artichokes
- Avocado
- Asparagus
- Broccoli
- Dates
- Beets
- Brussels sprouts
- Carrots
- Cabbage
- Cucumbers
- Cherries
- Figs
- Limes
- Mushrooms
- Melons
- Squash
- Spinach
- Pomegranate

Fish and meat

- Chicken
- Tuna

- Salmon
- Haddock
- Mackerel
- Turkey
- Mussels
- Shellfish
- Scallops
- Tilapia
- Clams
- Crab

Dairy and eggs

- Greek yogurt
- Low-fat milk
- Eggs
- Goat cheese
- Parmesan
- Mozzarella

CONCLUSION

I hope that at this point in the book, you are feeling a bit more confident about the Mediterranean diet. Remember that this isn't something you have to DIVE into. It is perfectly okay to plan on one meal for the week. This one meal is better than no meals at all. Slowly, you will become surer of your skills as you become able to prepare multiple meals in a week. Also, remember all of the incredible benefits that come with meal prepping!

If you take anything away, remember to choose a day and take the time. It may seem like you are spending a lot of time cooking, but remember that you will be saving that cooking and prepping time through your whole week. Now, you can focus on what you will spend all of this extra time doing! Perhaps, it will be taking that exercise class you have been thinking about or some quality family time. Either way, meal prepping can shed new light on a healthier lifestyle.

Hopefully, you have found at least one recipe within these chapters you are excited to try. Whether you are vegan, vegetarian, or eat everything, there is a recipe out there for you. As I said before, try to start simple.

Now, you know the Mediterranean diet is not just a dietary adjustment, but a complete change of lifestyle. Ancel Keys was the first to notice the link between the people of the Mediterranean's healthy heart diet and longer lifespan. In order to correctly emulate that, we must improve not only our diet but our physical activity as well. The people of the Mediterranean incorporated exercise into their routine regularly, and we must try and do the same. It doesn't have to be a set workout time at the gym, but rather taking a walk around the neighborhood or taking a long bike ride can help burn accumulated calories and spur weight loss. Weight loss can only occur if you are following a calorie deficit diet. Even if the Mediterranean diet is easy to follow in the sense that it doesn't require counting carbs or calories, it is still important that you are aware of your portion size if you want to lose weight. That can only happen if you are burning off more calories than what you are taking in!

So many diets fail because people focus on what they cannot eat. With the Mediterranean diet, there is a wider variety of food that you are allowed to eat! Though you should try and limit your dairy, red meat, and poultry intake because there are still many delicious meals you can prepare. You can still eat red meat or a chicken dish once a week, but try and use leaner cuts of meat and be conscious of your portion size. Incorporate more fish into your diet and have fresh fruits and vegetables on hand to create a quick salad. Also, remember that you should use extra virgin olive oil in your cooking and salad dressing. It is the basis for a healthy heart and are packed with antioxidants that keep your cells healthy and prevents inflammation in the body.

FINAL WORDS

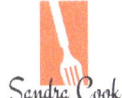

Finally, If you enjoyed this book and got helpful information, would you consider letting others know about it?

You can do it just leaving a review, or mention it to your friends, colleagues and family members.

Thank you!
 Sandra

MEASUREMENT CONVERSIONS

VOLUME EQUIVALENTS (LIQUID)

US Standard	US Standard (ounces)	Metric (approximate)
2 tablespoons	1 fl. oz.	30 mL
¼ cup	2 fl. oz.	60 mL
½ cup	4 fl. oz.	120 mL
1 cup	8 fl. oz.	240 mL
1½ cups	12 fl. oz.	355 mL
2 cups or 1 pint	16 fl. oz.	475 mL
4 cups or 1 quart	32 fl. oz.	1 L
1 gallon	128 fl. oz.	4 L

Volume Equivalents (Liquid)

OVEN TEMPERATURES

Fahrenheit (F)	Celsius (C) (approximate)
250°F	120°C
300°F	150°C
325°F	165°C
350°F	180°C
375°F	190°C

Oven Temperatures

400°F	200°C
425°F	220°C
450°F	230°C

Oven Temperatures

VOLUME EQUIVALENTS (DRY)

US Standard	Metric (approximate)
⅛ teaspoon	0.5 mL
¼ teaspoon	1 mL
½ teaspoon	2 mL
¾ teaspoon	4 mL
1 teaspoon	5 mL
1 tablespoon	15 mL
¼ cup	59 mL
⅓ cup	79 mL
½ cup	118 mL
⅔ cup	156 mL
¾ cup	177 mL
1 cup	235 mL
2 cups or 1 pint	475 mL
3 cups	700 mL

Volume Equivalents (Dry)

4 cups or 1 quart	1 L

Volume Equivalents (Dry)

WEIGHT EQUIVALENTS

US Standard	Metric (approximate)
½ ounce	15 g
1 ounce	30 g
2 ounces	60 g
4 ounces	115 g
8 ounces	225 g
12 ounces	340 g
16 ounces or 1 pound	455 g

Weight Equivalents

REFERENCES

Domínguez, L.J., M. Bes-Rastrollo, C. de la Fuente-Arrillaga, et al. "Similar prediction of decreased total mortality, diabetes incidence or cardiovascular events using relative and absolute-component Mediterranean diet score: The SUN cohort." **Nutrition, Metabolism and Cardiovascular Diseases**, March 6, 2012.

Estruch R., E. Ros, J. Salas-Salvadó, et al. "Primary prevention of cardiovascular disease with a Mediterranean diet." **The New England Journal of Medicine**, February 25, 2013.

Fernández-Real, J.M., M. Bulló, J.M. Moreno-Navarrete, et al. "A Mediterranean diet enriched with olive oil is associated with higher serum total osteocalcin levels in elderly men at high cardiovascular risk." **Journal of Clinical Endocrinology and Metabolism**, October 2012: 3792–98.

Gardener H., C.B. Wright, Y. Gu, et al. "Mediterranean-style diet and risk of ischemic stroke, myocardial infarction, and vascular death: the Northern Manhattan Study." **The American Journal of Clinical Nutrition**, vol. 94 no. 6 (December 2011): 1458–64.

Gil A., R.M. Ortega, J. Maldonado. "Wholegrain cereals and bread: a duet of the Mediterranean diet for the prevention of chronic diseases." **Public Health Nutrition**, 2011: 2316–22.

Haber B. "The Mediterranean Diet: a view from history." **The American Journal of Clinical Nutrition**, vol. 66 no. 4 (October 1997): 1053S–75.

Harvard School of Public Health. "Close adherence to a traditional Mediterranean diet promotes longevity." Press release, June 25, 2003. **http://archive.sph.harvard.edu/press-releases/archives/2003-releases/press06252003.html** (accessed March 20, 2013).

Kromhout D., A. Menotti, B. Bloemberg, et al. "Dietary saturated and trans fatty acids and cholesterol and 25-year mortality from coronary heart disease: the Seven Countries Study." **Preventive Medicine**, vol. 24 no. 3 (May 1995): 308–15.

Nordmann A. J., K. Suter-Zimmermann, H.C. Bucher, et al. "Meta-analysis comparing Mediterranean to low-fat diets for modification of cardiovascular risk factors." **The American Journal of Medicine**, vol. 124 no. 9 (September 2011): 841–51.

Scarmeas N., J. Luchsinger, R. Mayeaux, et al. "Mediterranean diet and Alzheimer disease mortality." **Neurology**, vol. 69 no. 11 (September 2007): 1084–93.

UNESCO.org. "Mediterranean diet," 2010. **http://www.unesco.org/culture/ich/en/RL/00394** (accessed March 20, 2012).

U.S. National Library of Medicine, National Institutes of Health. "Wine and heart health." MedLine Plus website, 2012. **http://www.nlm.nih.gov/medlineplus/ency/article/001963.htm** (accessed March 20, 2013).

Willet, W.C., F. Sacks, A. Trichopoulou, et al. "Mediterranean diet pyramid: a cultural model for healthy eating." **American Journal of Clinical Nutrition**, vol. 61 no. 6 (June 1995): 1402S–6S.

INDEX RECIPES

A

Awesome Ligurian Chicken 141

B

Baked Lamb with Eggplant and Greek Yogurt 105
    Baked Salmon in Garlic Pepper 159
    Baked Trout and Fennel 101
    Banana Nut Oatmeal 85
    Banana Strawberry Popsicles 211
    Beef Steaks with Spicy Sauce 108
    Breakfast Enchiladas 57
    Breakfast Quesadilla 45
    Buttery Carrot Sticks 238

C

Cajun Walnuts And Olives Bowls 240
    Carrot Slaw 299

Carrot Spread..230
Cayenne Cod and Tomatoes...127
Cheesy Mediterranean Scramble....................................67
Chia Almond Butter Pudding..215
Chicken And Broccoli Platter..185
Chicken and Cabbage Mix..177
Chicken Korma...192
Chicken Wings Platter..232
Chickpea & Potato Hash...53
Chili Calamari and Veggie Mix.....................................123
Chocolate Matcha Balls..213
Chocolate Mousse..227
Chocolate Mousse Dark..172
Cinnamon Baby Back Ribs Platter................................236
Classic Mediterranean Chicken Soup...........................172
Creamy Cuban Fu Fu..73
Creamy Loaded Mashed Potatoes..................................78
Creamy Yogurt Banana Bowls......................................225
Crunchy Roasted Chickpeas..201
Crisp Spiced Cauliflower with Feta Cheese.................256

D

Daring Salted Baked Chicken......................................188
   Delicious Chicken Soup..169
   Delicious Sausage Kebabs......................................111

E

Easy Chicken Stew...175
   Elbow Macaroni with Pine Nuts, Lemon and Fennel.....289

G

Garlic And Lemon Chicken Dish..................................144
   Garlic Shrimp with Olive Oil....................................149

Greek Frittata w/ Zucchini, Tomatoes, Feta, and Herbs......87
Greek Salad With Saganaki..301
Greek Scramble..65
Greek Trout Spread...125
Greek Yogurt Pancakes...90
Grilled Octopus...164

H

Healthy & Quick Energy Bites...223
    Healthy Coconut Blueberry Balls....................................199
    Healthy Mediterranean Chicken......................................181
    Hearty Breakfast Frittata w/ Tomato Salad.....................48
    High-Quality Belizean Chicken Stew..............................133
    Homemade Whole Wheat Pita Bread............................253
    Hot Asparagus Sticks...244
    Huevos Revueltos..71

L

Lemon Rice..297
    Lamb Steak Pita Breads..103
    Leeks and Calamari Mix...155
    Loaded Mediterranean Cauliflower Fries......................268

M

Magnificent Chicken Curry Soup..139
    Mango Salsa..242
    Mediterranean Breakfast Quinoa......................................55
    Mediterranean Breakfast Wraps..60
    Mediterranean Meatloaf...120
    Mediterranean Omelet...69
    Mediterranean Tofu Scramble...92
    Mediterranean-style Mussels...153
    Mushroom And Chicken Bowl.......................................183

Mediterranean Pasta Salad..261
Mediterranean Farro Salad..263
Mediterranean Couscous...266
Mediterranean Succotash..271
Mediterranean Couscous Salad...273
Mediterranean Barley Salad...276
Mediterranean Chicken Samosas with Apple Cumin C. ..283

P

Panera Mediterranean Breakfast Sandwich............................63
    Pork Bites..246
    Potato and Zucchini Omelet..80

R

Refreshing Strawberry Popsicles...217
    Roasted Almonds..209
    Roasted Asparagus Prosciutto & Egg................................75
    Roasted Green Beans...205

S

Salmon & Asparagus...131
    Salmon and Creamy Endives...99
    Sauteed Octopus..162
    Savory Pistachio Balls...207
    Scallop Salad...166
    Seafood Paella..157
    Secret Breakfast Sundaes..83
    Shrimp and Dill Mix..129
    Slow Cooked Chicken...117
    Smoked Salmon and Veggies Mix....................................97
    Spaghetti Frittata..50
    Steamed Mussels in Tomato Garlic.................................151
    Stuffed Chicken..234

Saffron Rice Salad..295
Spinach Salad with Grilled Mediterranean Vegetables......281
Spring Peas and Beans with Zesty Thyme Yogurt Sauce...258

T

Tabbouleh...279
    Tasty Zucchini Chips..203
    Tender Roasted Sweet Potatoes with Savory Tahini S.......251
    The Great Poblano Chicken Curry..................................135
    The Original Mexican Chicken Cacciatore.....................137
    Turkey Cutlets...90
    Turkey With Garlic Sauce..114
    Toasted Israeli Couscous with Vegetables.......................286

V

Vegetable Couscous...292

W

Warm & Soft Baked Pears..221
    Worthy Ghee-Licious Chicken 190

www.ingramcontent.com/pod-product-compliance
Lightning Source LLC
Chambersburg PA
CBHW071217080526
44587CB00013BA/1402